WEIGHT LOSS FC

SHREDDING THE POUNDS, THE FEMALE WAY

The Ultimate Intermittent Fasting For Women With Workout, Diet, And Meal Plans To Achieve A Great Body

ADELYN NEWTON

Table of Contents

PART I

Introduction

Be gentle with yourself throughout this process as it will be uncomfortable at times and will require strength. This book will help you through it, as you are not alone. I hope that this book also reminds you that many other people are suffering from the same type of food-related disorders as you are and that you are not alone in that either. This book will take a step-by-step approach, which will make for the highest chance of recovery. If at any time you need to take a break in order to think about the information you have learned, feel free to do so, but make sure you come back to this book quite soon after. Going through this process of recovery can be a lot, but with the right support, it will be possible.

You have already taken the first step in recovery, which is acknowledging that you have an issue. For that, I congratulate you!

What Is Emotional Eating?

Emotional eating occurs when a person suffering from emotional deficiencies of some sort, including lack of affection, lack of connection, or other factors like stress, depression, anxiety, or even general negative feelings like sadness or anger, eats in order to gain comfort from the food they are eating.

Many people find comfort in food. When people experience negative feelings and turn to food consumption in order to reduce their pain or to feel better, this is called emotional eating.

Now, some people do this on occasion like after a breakup or after a bad fight, but when this occurs at least a few times a week, this is when it is considered to have a negative impact on one's life and is when it becomes an issue that needs to be addressed.

What Is Binge Eating?

Binge eating disorder is another disorder that can be seen along with emotional eating. Binge eating disorder is when a person eats much more than a regular amount of food in a single occasion or sitting, and they feel unable to control themselves or to stop themselves. This could also be defined as a compulsion to overeat. In order to be considered a disorder, it has to happen at least two times per week for longer than six months consecutively.

Along with binge eating is overeating, although this is also sometimes seen as a separate disorder altogether. Overeating is when a person eats more than they require in order to sustain life. This occurs when they consume much more than they need in a day, or in a single sitting.

Overeating does not necessarily become binge eating, but it certainly can. Overeating is a general term used to describe the eating disorders that we just defined-Emotional Eating and Binge Eating. Thus, overeating could involve binge eating, food addiction, or other food-related disorders.

In this book, we will be focusing on emotional eating and binge eating, and how you can overcome these two food-related disorders.

What Is Bulimia?

Bulimia is another eating disorder. Bulimia involves binge eating, followed by extreme feelings of shame, guilt, and disdain for oneself and one's body. This is accompanied by intense feelings of body dysmorphia and body image issues, as well as the desire to be "skinnier." Thus, the person will turn to purging- or self-inflicted vomiting in an effort to lose weight and rid themselves of the guilt and shame.

Chapter 1: Understanding Your Food-Related Disorder

In this chapter, we are going to look at these two food-related disorders (binge eating/ bulimia and emotional eating) in much more detail. We will begin by looking at the most common reasons why people suffer from these disorders and will spend some time examining scientific research about why these disorders exist.

Why Do People Eat Emotionally?

The reason that emotional eating occurs is that eating foods that we enjoy makes us feel rewarded on an emotional and physiological level within our brain.

Why Do People Binge Eat?

People binge eat for a very similar reason to the reason why people experience emotional eating. This is because eating foods that we enjoy in terms of taste, smell, texture, and so on, makes us feel rewarded on an emotional and physiological level within our brains.

Throughout the rest of this chapter, we will look more in-depth at these eating disorders in order to give you more information about why they occur and what could cause them.

Scientific Research on Eating Disorders and Why They Exist

You may be asking how food cravings can result from emotional deficiencies and how these two seemingly unrelated things can be considered related. While we have touched on this briefly in this book already, the reason for this is that your body learns, over time, that eating certain foods makes it feel rewarding, positive, and happy for some time after it is ingested. These foods include convenience foods such as those containing processed sugars or salts, fast food, and quick pastries.

When you are sad or worried, your body feels negative and looks for ways to remedy this. Your brain then connects these two facts- that the body does not feel positive and that it wants to find a way to fix this. The brain then decides that eating the foods that make it feel good will remedy the situation. This process happens in the background of your mind without you being aware of it, and it leads you to consciously feel a craving for those specific foods such as sugary snacks or salty fast-food meals. You may not even be aware of why. If you then decide to give in to this craving and eat something like a microwave pizza snack, your body will feel rewarded and happy for a brief period of time. This reinforces to your brain that turning to food in an effort to make yourself feel better emotionally has been successful.

If you end up feeling down and guilty that you ate something that was unhealthy or that you ate too much, your brain will again try and remedy these negative emotions by craving food. This is how a cycle of emotional eating or a cycle of bingeing and purging can begin and continue. This could happen largely in your subconscious without you being any the wiser.

Why Do People Have Bulimia or Other Food Disorders?

Because scientists and psychiatrists understand this process that occurs in the brain, they know that food cravings can indicate emotional deficiencies. While there are other types of cravings that can occur, such as those that pregnant ladies experience, or those that indicate nutrient deficiencies, there are ways to tell that a craving is caused by some type of emotional deficiency.

It begins by determining the foods that a person craves and when they crave them. If every time someone has a stressful situation, they feel like eating a pizza, or if a person who is depressed tends to eat a lot of chocolate, this could indicate emotional eating. As you know by now, emotional eating and bulimia are closely related, and emotional eating can lead to bulimia over time.

If you crave fruit like a watermelon on a hot day, you are likely just dehydrated, and your body is trying to get water from a water-filled fruit that it knows will make it more hydrated. Examining situations like this has led scientists and psychiatrists to explore eating disorders in more depth and determine what types of emotional deficiencies can manifest themselves through food cravings or disordered eating in this way.

In the next chapter, we will look at psychological triggers that can lead to disordered eating.

The Neuroscience of Brain Chemicals and Food As a Reward

Many times, we may see ingredients on the packages of foods we eat, but we aren't really sure of exactly what they are, just that they taste good. In this section, we will take a deeper look at them and what they do to your brain.

Casein is a heavily processed ingredient that is derived from milk. It is processed a few times over and eventually creates milk solids that are concentrated. These milk solids- called Casein are then added into foods like cheese, french fries, milkshakes, and other fast and convenient packaged or fast-foods that contain dairy or dairy products (such as pastries and salad dressings). Casein has been compared to nicotine in its addictive properties. It is often seen in cheese, and this is why there is increasing evidence that people can become, and many are already addicted to cheese. The reason for this is during digestion. When cheese and other foods that contain casein are digested, it is broken down, and one of the compounds that it breaks down into is a compound that is strikingly similar to opioids- the highly addictive substance that is in pain killers.

High fructose corn syrup is surely an ingredient you have heard of before or at least one that you have seen on the packaging of your favorite snacks or quick foods. While this is actually derived from real corn, after it is finished being processed, there is nothing corn-like about it. High fructose corn syrup is essentially the same thing as refined sugar when all is said and done. It is used as a sweetener in foods like soda, cereal, and other sweet and quick foods. The reason why this ingredient is seen so often is that it is much cheaper than using sugar and is much easier to work with. High Fructose Corn Syrup is another common food additive that has been shown to be highly addictive. This substance has been shown to be similar to cocaine in its addictive properties.

MSG stands for Monosodium Glutamate, which sounds a lot like a chemical you may have encountered in science class in college. MSG is added to foods to give it a delicious flavor. It is essentially a very concentrated form of salt. What this does in foods such as fast-food, packaged convenience foods, and buffet-style food is that it gives it that wonderfully salty and fatty flavor that makes us keep coming back for more. Companies put this in food because it comes at an extremely low cost, and the flavor it brings covers up the artificial flavors of all of the other cheap ingredients that are used to make these foods. MSG has been known to block our natural appetite suppressant, which normally kicks in when we have had enough to eat. For this reason, when we are eating foods containing MSG, we do not recognize when we are satiated, and we continue to eat until we are stuffed because it tastes so great.

Chapter 2: Understanding Your Mind

In this chapter, we are going to look at some of the psychological factors that can lead to disordered eating so that you can gain a better understanding of what could have led you to use food as a means of coping.

Psychological and Emotional Triggers

There are several types of emotional deficiencies that can be indicated by disordered eating. We will explore these in detail below in hopes that you will recognize some of the reasons why you may be struggling with an eating disorder.

Childhood Causes

The first example of an emotional deficiency that we will examine is more of an umbrella for various emotional deficiencies. This umbrella term is Childhood Causes. If you think back on your childhood, think about how your relationship with food was cultivated. Maybe you were taught that when you behaved, you received food as a reward. Maybe when you were feeling down, you were given food to cheer you up. Maybe you turned to food when you were experiencing negative things in your childhood. Any of these could cause someone to suffer from emotional eating in their adulthood, as it had become something learned. This type is quite difficult to break as it has likely been a habit for many, many years, but it is possible. When we are children, we learn habits and make associations without knowing it that we often carry into our later lives. While this is no fault of yours, recognizing it as a potential issue is important to make changes.

Covering Up Emotions

Another emotional deficiency that can manifest itself in emotional eating and food cravings is actually the effort to cover up our emotions. Sometimes we would rather distract ourselves and cover up our emotions than to feel them or to face them head-on. In this case, our brain may make us feel hungry in an effort to distract us from the act of eating food. When we have a quiet minute where these feelings or thoughts would pop into our minds, we can cover them up by deciding to prepare food and eat and convince ourselves that we are "too busy" to acknowledge our feelings because we have to deal with our hunger. The fact that it is hunger that arises in this scenario makes it very difficult to ignore and very easy to deem as a necessary distraction since, after all, we do need to eat in order to survive. This can be a problem though, if we are not in need of nourishment, and we are telling ourselves that this is the reason why we cannot deal with our demons or our emotions. If there is something that you think you may be avoiding dealing with or thinking about or if you tend to be very uncomfortable with feelings of unrest, you may be experiencing this type of emotional eating.

Feeling Empty or Bored

When we feel bored, we often decide to eat or decide that we are hungry. This occupies our mind and our time and makes us feel less bored and even feel positive and happy. We also may eat when we are feeling empty. When we feel empty the food will quite literally be ingested in an effort to fill a void, but as we know, the food will not fill a void that is emotional in sort, and this will lead to an unhealthy cycle of trying to fill ourselves emotionally with something that will never actually work. This will lead us to become disappointed every time and continue trying to fill this void with material things like food or purchases. This can also be a general feeling of dissatisfaction with life and feelings of lacking something in your life. Looking deeper into this the next time you feel those cravings will be difficult but will help you greatly in the long term as you will then be able to identify the source of your feelings of emptiness and begin to fill these voids in ways that will be much more effective.

Affection Deficiency

Another emotional deficiency that could manifest itself as food cravings is an affection deficiency. This type of deficiency can be feelings of loneliness, feelings of a lack of love, or feelings of being undesired. If a person has been without an intimate relationship or has recently gone through a breakup, or if a person has not experienced physical intimacy in quite some time, they may be experiencing an affection deficiency. This type of emotional deficiency will often manifest itself in food cravings as we will try to gain feelings of comfort and positivity from the good tasting, drug-like (as we talked about in chapter one) foods they crave.

Low Self-Esteem

Another emotional deficiency that may be indicated by food cravings is a low level of self-esteem. Low self-esteem can cause people to feel down, unlovable, inadequate, and overall negative and sad. This can make a person feel like eating foods they enjoy will make them feel better, even if only for a few moments. Low self-esteem is an emotional deficiency that is difficult to deal with as it affects every area of a person's life, such as their love life, their social life, their career life, and so on. Sometimes people have reported feeling like food was something that was always there for them, and that never left them. While this is true, they will often be left feeling even emptier and lower about themselves after giving into cravings.

Mood

A general low mood can cause emotional eating. While the problem of emotional eating is something that is occurring multiple times per week and we all have general low moods or bad days, if this makes you crave food and especially food of an unhealthy sort, this could become emotional eating. If every time we feel down or are having a bad day, we want to eat food to make ourselves feel better; this is emotional eating. Some people will have a bad day and want a drink at the end of the day, and if this happens every once in a while, it is not necessarily a problem with emotional eating. The more often it happens, the more often it is emotional eating. Further, we do not have to give in to the cravings for it to be considered emotional eating. Experiencing the cravings often and in tandem with negative feelings in the first place is what constitutes emotional eating.

Depression

Suffering from depression also can lead to emotional eating. Depression is a constant low mood for a period of months on end, and this low mood can cause a person to turn to food for comfort and a lift in spirit. This can then become emotional eating in addition to and because of depression.

Anxiety

Having anxiety can lead to emotional eating, as well. There are several types of anxiety, and whether it is general anxiety (constant levels of anxiety), situational anxiety (triggered by a situation or scenario), it can lead to emotional eating. You have likely heard of the term *comfort food* to describe certain foods and dishes. The reason for this is because they are usually foods rich in carbohydrates, fats, and heavy in nature. These foods bring people a sense of comfort. These foods are often turned to when people suffering from anxiety are emotionally eating because these foods help to temporarily ease their anxiety and make them feel calmer and more at ease. This only lasts for a short period of time; however, before their anxiety usually gears up again.

Stress

Stress eating is probably the most common form of emotional eating. While this does not become an issue for everyone experiencing stress, and many people will do so every once in a while, it is a problem for those who consistently turn to food to ease their stress. Some people are always under stress, and they will constantly be looking for ways to ease their stress. Food is one of these ways that people use to make themselves feel better and to take their minds off of their stress. As with all of the other examples we have seen above, this is not a lasting resolution, and it becomes a cycle. Similar to the cycle diagram we saw above, the same can be used for stress except instead of a negative emotion and eating making you feel more down, stress eating can make you feel more stress as you feel like you have done something you shouldn't have which causes you stress, and the cycle ensues.

Recognizing your triggers is important because this will allow you to notice when you may be feeling emotional hunger and when you are feeling actual hunger. If you become hungry, you can look back on your day or on the last hour and determine if any of your triggers were present. If they were, then you will be able to determine that you are likely experiencing emotional hunger, and you can take the appropriate steps instead of giving in to the cravings blindly.

There are many different emotional causes for the cravings we experience. There may be others than those listed above, and these are all valid. A person's emotional eating experience is unique and personal and could be caused by any number of things. You may also experience a combination of emotional deficiencies listed above, or one of those listed above in addition to others. Many of these can overlap, such as anxiety and depression, which are often seen together in a single person. The level of these emotional deficiencies that you experience could indicate the level of emotional eating that you struggle with. Whatever your experience and your struggles though, there is hope of recovery, and this is what the rest of this book will focus on.

Chapter 3: How to Stop Binge Eating, Bulimia, and Emotional Eating

In this chapter, we are going to look at how you can begin to tackle your mind in order to make positive changes for your body and break free from your eating disorder once and for all.

Addressing the Core Wounds

The key to solving these food-related issues is to address your core wounds. Understanding how your mind works will help you to better take care of it. You will be able to recognize your feelings and how they could have come about, and then treat them in a way that will help it to feel better. Bettering your relationship with food and your body will also improve your relationship with your mind. This will then allow you to begin to feed it what it needs, which will, in turn, lead to better cognitive functioning, control over impulses, and decision-making. This will help overall in your relationship with your food, your body, and your mind.

What Are Core Wounds?

As we discussed in the previous chapter, there are several types of emotional deficiencies that can be indicated by disordered eating. Once you have determined which of these emotional deficiencies (or which combination of them) are present in your life, you can begin to look at them in a little more detail. By doing so, you will come upon your core wounds. A core wound is something that you believe to be true about yourself or your life, and it is something that likely came about as a result of a coping mechanism you developed to deal with childhood. For example, this could be something like; the feeling of not being enough, the belief that you are unlovable, or the belief that you are stupid.

How to Address Them

By understanding and addressing your core wounds, you will be able to change your behaviors because of the intricate relationship that exists between your thoughts, your emotions, and your behaviors. By addressing your thoughts and emotions, you will change your behaviors and thus, free yourself from disordered eating. You may be wondering how you can begin to address your core wounds, as it can be difficult to know where to begin.

The first step is learning how to control and change your thoughts, which in turn, leads to changes in your behavior. By taking control of your thoughts and your beliefs, they don't have the opportunity to manifest into unhealthy behaviors such as overeating, turning to food for comfort, or any other unhealthy coping mechanisms that you have developed over the course of your life.

Becoming aware of your own thoughts is the most crucial step in this entire guide, as everything else will fail without it. Paying attention to your thoughts will help you identify what thoughts are going through your mind during an intense emotional moment. By looking deep within, in order to get in touch with your deepest feelings, you will be more likely to succeed in your weight loss and your overall lifestyle improvement.

One great example of how to put this into practice is through the use of journaling. Journaling can help in a process such as this because it can help you to organize your thoughts and feelings and will help you to see visually what is working and what isn't working for you. While we can give tips and examples, every person is different, so to find exactly what works for you, you will have to try some different things and see which techniques help you personally the most and in the best way. Journaling can be about anything like how you feel since beginning a new program, how you feel physically since changing your diet, how you feel emotionally now that you are not reaching for food in order to comfort your emotions and anything along the lines of this.

Positive Self-Talk

Once you have addressed your emotions and your core wounds, you can begin to intervene and change them so that they result in healthier behaviors. You will do this using positive self-talk. Adopting helpful thought processes fosters better emotions overall, which leads to more productive behaviors.

When people have developed unhelpful thinking processes, it is hard to make decisions to benefit their future selves because their thoughts create negative emotions that drive away motivation. This is where something called *positive self-talk* can come in. Positive self-talk can be instrumental in helping you to recover from disordered eating.

What Is Positive Self-Talk?

Many people's minds are controlled by their inner critic. The inner critic shares words with you, such as "You should just give up" Or "What makes you think you'll succeed?" which is rooted in the opposite of positive self-talk- Negative self-talk!

Instead of creating an open space that allows for mistakes, growth, and development, your inner critic causes you to question your worth, which makes it difficult for you to have the positive, growth mindset that is needed to complete tasks and go after things that may be difficult to achieve. In this case, helping your mind to begin using positive self-talk will help you to recover for the long-term.

How to Use Positive Self-Talk?

Below are several ways that you can begin to use positive self-talk. Over time, your mind will get used to thinking in this way, and you will find it much easier to do.

1. Remind yourself

Bad habits are built through many years, and no amount of willpower can undo a lifetime of bad habits, such as a strong inner critic that uses negative self-talk. By rewiring your brain to minimize the amount of negativity you feel in the first place, you will eventually get used to filling your mind with positive thoughts instead of negative ones.

2. Stop the automatic process of negativity

Often times, if the person had just paid attention to their thought process, they would be able to catch themselves before their mind automatically spiraled to a place of complete de-motivation. By catching yourself before you get there, you can prevent yourself from falling into your negative thought patterns that are limiting you and holding you back.

3. Find positive influences

Surrounding yourself with people that can encourage you and foster positivity will also change your inner-critic's opinion. Often times, hearing positive compliments from other people hold a heavier weight in the eyes of your inner-critic compared to you telling your inner-critic the same thing. Try spending time with people who are supportive of your goals and the changes that you are looking to make in your life. It will make your journey a little bit easier.

4. Limit Negative Influences

By limiting the negative influences in your life, you are making a statement to yourself that you place importance on preserving your mental health. When you remove negative influences and limit your exposure to things or people that make you feel negative, you are prioritizing yourself, and this is a great way to practice self-care.

5. Practice a gratitude exercise

This is a great exercise to remind yourself of everything that you love and appreciate about yourself and your life. Take time to write down all of the things that you love about yourself and about your life. This will remind you of all of the positivity surrounding you and will serve to uplift you.

Chapter 4: Making Healthier Decisions Using Intuitive

Eating

This chapter will provide you with a solid foundation of knowledge on which to build your new lifestyle. We will look at how intuitive eating can be the answer to all of your struggles and help you to find recovery.

Making Good Choices

As we discussed in the previous chapter, making good choices begins with self-exploration and a deep look into your core wounds. Once you have done this, you can begin to make decisions that are positive for your health and your life, and over time these will become more and more habitual. We are going to spend this chapter looking at some of the ways that you can begin to make good choices related to food and eating.

How to Begin Making Good Choices Using Intuitive Eating

One great way to make good choices when it comes to food is by using something called intuitive eating. Below, I will define intuitive eating for you and give you some insight into how this can change your life.

What Is Intuitive Eating?

Intuitive eating is a new perspective from which to view how you feed your body. This style of eating puts you in control, instead of following a list of pre-designed guidelines about when and what to eat. Intuitive eating instead encourages you to listen to your body and the signals it sends you about what, how much, and when to eat. This ensures that you are giving your body exactly what it needs when it needs it, instead of forcing it into a specific kind of diet.

Intuitive eating does not limit any specific foods and does not require you to stick to certain foods exclusively. Instead, it encourages you to learn as much as you can about what your body is telling you and follow its signals.

The two main components of the intuitive eating philosophy are the following; eat when you are hungry and stop eating when you are satiated. This may seem like a no-brainer, but in today's societies, we are very far from eating in an intuitive way, as odd as it may seem. With so many diet trends and numerous "rules" for how you should and should not eat, it can be difficult to put these ideas aside and let your body guide you exclusively.

Intuitive Eating and Hunger

Before we begin looking at the specifics of intuitive eating, we will look at the different types of hunger and how you can tell them apart. This will help you to distinguish when you are hungry and when you may be turning to food to soothe your emotional state.

Real hunger is when our body needs nutrients or energy and is letting us know that we should replenish our energy soon. This happens when it has been a few hours since our last meal when we wake up in the morning, or after a lot of strenuous activity like a long hike. Our body uses hunger to signal to us that it is in need of more energy and that if it doesn't get it soon, it will begin to use our stored energy as fuel. While there is nothing wrong with our body using its stored fuel, it can be used as a sign to us that we should eat shortly in order to replenish these stores. Perceived Hunger is when we think we are hungry, but our body doesn't actually require any more energy or for the stores to be replenished. This can happen for a number of reasons, including an emotional deficiency, a negative mental state, or the occurrence of a psychological trigger.

The philosophy behind intuitive eating is that if you wait until you are too hungry before eating, you will be much more likely to overeat or to binge eat. This is because, by this time, you be feeling ravenous instead of mildly hungry. If instead, you choose to adhere to your hunger and eat when your body tells you that it needs sustenance, you will be much more likely to eat just the right amount. As a result, your body will be satisfied rather than completely stuffed, and instead of feeling shameful and angry that you have eaten, you can feel happy that you have provided your body with what it needed. This requires you to listen to and respect what your body is telling you and then provide it with nutrients in order for it to keep working hard for you!

The Benefits of Intuitive Eating

One of the reasons that intuitive eating is such a successful and cherished form of eating is that it allows the body to lead the mind in the right direction when it comes to seeking out its needs. Below, we will look at the benefits of letting your body guide your eating choices.

- Allows the body to get what it needs

Did you know that your cravings could actually be giving you much more information than you give them credit for?

A craving is an intense longing for something (in this case food), that comes about intensely and feels urgent. In our case, that longing is for s a very specific type of food. When we have cravings for certain foods, it can actually mean more than what it seems.

While you may think that a craving is an indication of hunger or of a desire for the taste of a certain food, it may actually indicate that your body is low on certain vitamins or minerals. As a result, your body seeks out a certain food that it thinks will provide it with this vitamin or mineral. This reaches your consciousness in the form of an intense craving. In this case, the body is trying to help itself by telling you what to eat. For this reason, understanding your cravings could help you give your body exactly what it is longing for.

For example, if you are craving juice or pop or other sugary drinks like this, consider that you might actually be dehydrated and, therefore, thirsty. Sometimes we see drinks in our fridge, and since we are thirsty, we really want them. Next time you are craving a sugary drink, try having a glass of water first, then wait a few minutes and see if you are still craving that Coca-Cola. You may not want it anymore once your thirst is quenched.

If you are craving meat, you may feel like you want some fried chicken or a hot dog. This can indicate a deficit of iron or protein. The best sources of protein are chicken breast cooked in the oven, and iron is best received from spinach, oysters, or lentils. If you think you may not like these foods, there are many different ways to prepare them, and you can likely find a way that you like.

- Prevents overeating

It can be hard to know how much to eat and when you have had enough to eat without letting yourself eat too much. Sometimes people will eat until the point that they begin to feel completely full. Many times, we keep eating until we become stuffed, even to the point of making ourselves feel physically ill. Intuitive eating will help you to avoid this, as this kind of eating encourages you to give your body what it needs in order to take great care of it. Stuffing your body until it is too full is not what your body is asking for, and once you become accustomed to listening to your body's needs, you will know when it is time to stop.

- Helps you break free from self-judgment

intuitive eating will help you to finally make peace with your body and yourself as a whole. It does this by showing you that your body has needs and that there is no shame in tending to these needs, as long as you do so in a healthy way.

You cannot fully embrace and practice intuitive eating if you have those nagging feelings of self-judgment each time you take a bite of food or decide that you are going to eat lunch when you are hungry. For this reason, in order to practice intuitive eating, you must understand that feeding your body is an act of compassion for yourself and that this does not need to come with self-judgment.

- It is inclusive, not exclusive

One of the great things about this style of eating is that it is not founded on restricting a person's intake of certain foods or allowing only a small variety of foods.

Diets like this are extremely hard to transition to and are hard to maintain for a long period of time. Intuitive eating is about including as many natural whole foods as you wish, while also ensuring that you are consuming enough of all of your nutrients. With this style of eating, you can eat whatever you wish, whenever you wish. This makes it much easier to stick with this type of diet and reduces the chances of falling off after a short period of time due to cravings or intense hunger. It does not restrict calories or reduce your intake greatly, which makes it easier to handle than a traditional diet for many people. It feels natural to eat in this way, which makes it effective.

Chapter 5: Intuitive Eating Part 2

In this chapter, we are going to continue our examination of intuitive eating by looking at some more specific details related to this diet, as well as how to make it a regular part of your life.

How to Make Intuitive Eating Part of Your Life

One of the best ways to make this type of eating a part of your life is to practice it with intention. This is especially important when you are just beginning. Each time you feel a pang of hunger or a compulsion to eat, take a minute to examine your inner world. By doing this, you will get your mind and body accustomed to working together. In addition, do the same after you eat. By doing these two things, you will be able to ensure that you are eating when hungry and stopping when satisfied.

When you finish eating a meal, rank your level of fullness on a scale of 1 to 10, 1 being extremely hungry and 10 being extremely stuffed. This will help you to determine if you are successfully stopping when you are satisfied and not overeating.

It is also important that you learn how to deal with your emotions and feelings in an effective way without using food. Using the techniques that you have learned in this book, you will be able to address your inner demons, which will make space for you to listen to your body and its needs.

As you know by now, listening to your body, your emotions and your mind is extremely important when it comes to practicing intuitive eating. As long as you remember this, you will be well on your way to becoming a lifelong intuitive eater.

What Kind of Foods Should You Choose?

Fish is a great way to get healthy fats into your diet. Certain fish are very low in carbohydrates but high in good fats, making them perfect for a healthy diet. They also contain minerals and vitamins that will be good for your health. Salmon is a great fish to eat, as it is versatile and delicious. Many fish also include essential fatty acids that we can only get through our diet. Other fish that are good for you include:

- Sardines
- Mackerel
- Herring
- Trout
- Albacore Tuna

Meat and Poultry make up a large part of most Americans' diets. Meats and poultry that are fresh and not processed do not include any carbohydrates and contain high levels of protein. Eating lean meats helps to maintain your strength and muscle mass and gives you energy for hours. Grass-fed meats, in particular, are rich in antioxidants.

Eggs are another amazing, protein-filled food. Eggs help your body to feel satiated for longer and also keeps your blood sugar levels consistent, which is great for overall health. The whole egg is good for you, as the yolk is where the nutrients are. The cholesterol found within egg yolks also has been demonstrated to lower your risk of getting diseases like heart diseases, despite what most people think. Therefore, do not be afraid of the egg yolk!

Legumes are a great source of protein as well as fiber, and there are many different types to choose from. These include the following:

- All sorts of beans including black beans, green beans, and kidney beans
- Peas
- Lentils of all colors
- Chickpeas
- Peas

Examples of fruits that you can eat include the following:

- Citrus fruits such as oranges, grapefruits, lemons, and limes
- Melons of a variety of sorts
- Apples
- Bananas
- Berries including strawberries, blueberries, blackberries, raspberries and so on
- Grapes

Vegetables are a great source of energy and nutrients, and they include a wide range of naturally occurring vivid colors which should all be included in your diet.

- Carrots
- Broccoli and cauliflower

- Asparagus
- Kale
- All sorts of peppers including hot peppers, bell peppers
- Tomatoes
- Root vegetables (that are a good source of healthy, complete carbohydrates) such as potatoes, sweet potatoes, all types of squash, and beets.

Seeds are another great source of nutrients, vitamins, and minerals, and they are very versatile. These include the following:

- Sesame seeds
- Pumpkin seeds
- Sunflower seeds
- Hemp, flax and chia seeds are all especially good for your health

Nuts are a great way to get protein if you are choosing not to eat meat or if you are vegan. They also are packed with nutrients. Some examples are below.

- Almonds
- Brazil Nuts
- Cashews
- Macadamia nuts
- Pistachios
- Pecans

There are some **healthy fats** that are essential components of any person's diet, as the beneficial compounds that they contain cannot be made by our bodies; thus, we rely solely on or diet to get them. These compounds are Omega-3 Fatty

Acids, monounsaturated and polyunsaturated fats. Below are some healthy sources of these compounds:

- Avocados
- Healthy, plant-based oils including olive oil and canola oil
- Hemp, chia and flax seeds
- Walnuts

When it comes to carbohydrates, these should be consumed in the form of **whole grains**, as they are high in fiber, which will help to prevent overeating. Whole grains also include essential minerals- those that we can only get from our diet just like those essential compounds found in healthy fats. These essential minerals are selenium, magnesium, and copper. Sources of these whole grains include the following:

- Quinoa
- Rye, Barley, buckwheat
- Whole grain oats
- Brown rice
- Whole grain bread can be hard to find these days in the grocery store, as many brown breads disguise themselves as whole grain when, in fact, they are not. However, there are whole grain breads if you take the time to look at the ingredients list.

Nutrients You Need and How to Get Them

In this section, we are going to look at the most beneficial nutrients for your body and where/ how you can find them. This will help you to decide which foods to include in your diet so that you can ensure you are getting all of the nutrients that your body needs.

1. Omega-3 Fatty Acids

Some vitamins and nutrients are called "essential nutrients." Omega-3 Fatty Acids are an example of this type of nutrient. They are called essential nutrients because they cannot be made by our bodies; thus, they must be eaten in our diets. These fatty acids are a very specific type of fatty acid, and this type, in particular, is the most essential and the most beneficial for our brains and bodies.

They have numerous effects on the brain, including reducing inflammation (which reduces the risk of Alzheimer's) and maintaining and improving mood and cognitive function, including specifically memory. Omega-3's have these greatly beneficial effects because of the way that they act in the brain, which is what makes them so essential to our diets. Omega-3 Fatty Acids increase the production of new nerve cells in the brain by acting specifically on the nerve stem cells within the brain, causing new and healthy nerve cells to be generated.

Omega-3 fatty acids can be found in fish like salmon, sardines, black cod, and herring. It can also be taken as a pill-form supplement for those who do not eat fish or cannot eat enough of it. It can also be taken in the form of a fish oil supplement like krill oil.

Omega-3 is by far the most important nutrient that you need to ensure you are ingesting because of the numerous benefits that come from it, both in the brain and in the rest of the body. While supplements are often a last step when it comes to trying to include something in your diet, for Omega-3's, the benefits are too great to potentially miss by trying to receive all of it from your diet.

Magnesium

Magnesium is beneficial for your diet, as it also helps you to maintain strong bones and teeth. Magnesium and Calcium are most effective when ingested together, as Magnesium helps in the absorption of calcium. It also helps to reduce migraines and is great for calmness and relieving anxiety. Magnesium can be found in leafy green vegetables like kale and spinach, as well as fruits like bananas and raspberries, legumes like beans and chickpeas, vegetables like peas, cabbage, green beans, asparagus, and brussels sprouts, and fish like tuna and salmon.

Calcium

Calcium is beneficial for the healthy circulation of blood, and for maintaining strong bones and teeth. Calcium can come from dairy products like milk, yogurt, and cheese. It can also be found in leafy greens like kale and broccoli and sardines.

Chapter 6: How to Make These New Choices a Habit

Now that you have learned a wealth of information about intuitive eating, we are going to look at some strategies that you can use to make these new, healthy choices a habit. This will take time, but by employing these strategies, you will surely find success.

Healthy Thinking Patterns

In this section, we will look at a real-life example of dealing with challenges to demonstrate healthy thinking patters when it comes to intuitive eating.

Let's say you are trying to focus on healthy eating, and you find that you have had trouble doing so. Maybe you ate a cupcake, or maybe you had a soda at breakfast. From the perspective of traditional diet mentality, this would become a problem for the diet, and this would become a problem in your mind as well. You would likely be beating yourself up and feeling terrible about the choice you have made.

Let's look at this example in more detail. It is very important to avoid beating yourself up or self-judging for falling off the wagon. This may happen sometimes. What we need to do though, is to focus not on the fact that it has happened, but on how we are going to deal with and react to it. There are a variety of reactions that a person may have to this type of situation. We will examine the possible reactions and their pros and cons below:

- You may feel as though your progress is ruined and that you might as well begin again another time. This could lead you to go back to your old ways and keep you from trying again for quite some time. This could happen many times, over and over again, and each time you slip up, you decide that you might as well give up this time and try again, but each time it ends the same.

- You may fall off of your plan and tell yourself that this day is a write-off and that you will begin again the next day. The problem with this method is that continuing the rest of the day as you would have before you decided to make a change will make it so that the next day is like beginning all over again, and it will be very hard to begin again. You may be able to begin again the next day, and it could be fine, but you must be able to really motivate yourself if you are going to do this. Knowing that you have fallen off before makes it so that you may feel down on yourself and feel as though you can't do it, so beginning again the next day is very important.

- The third option, similar to the previous case, you may fall off, but instead of deciding that the day is a write-off, you tell yourself that the entire week is a write-off, and you then decide that you will pick it up again the next week. This will be even harder than starting again the next day as multiple days of eating whatever you like will make it very hard to go back to making the healthy choices again afterward.

- After eating something that you wish you hadn't (and that wasn't a healthy choice), you decide not to eat anything for the rest of the day so that you don't eat too many calories or too much sugar, and decide that the next day you will start over again. This is very difficult on the body as you are going to be quite hungry by the time the evening rolls around. Instead of forgiving yourself, you are punishing yourself, and it will make it very hard not to reach for chips late at night when you are starving and feeling down.

- The fifth and final option is what you should do in this situation.

This option is the best for success and will make it the most likely that you will succeed long-term. If you fall off at lunch, let's say, because you are tired and, in a rush, and you just grab something from a fast-food restaurant instead of going home for lunch or buying something at the grocery store to eat, this is how we will deal with it. Firstly, you will likely feel like you have failed and may feel quite down about having made an unhealthy choice. Now instead of starving for the rest of the day or eating only lettuce for dinner, you will put this slip up at lunch behind you, and you will continue your day as if it never happened. You will eat a healthy dinner as you planned, and you will continue on with the plan. You will not wait until tomorrow to begin again; you will continue as you would if you had made that healthy choice at lunch. The key to staying on track is being able to bounce back. The people who can bounce back mentally are the ones who will be most likely to succeed. You will need to maintain a positive mental state and look forward to the rest of the day and the rest of the week in just the same way as you did before you had a slip-up. One bad meal out of the entire week is not going to ruin all of your progress and recovering from emotional eating is largely a mental game. It is more mental than anything else, so we must not underestimate the role that our mindset plays in our success or failure.

By using this type of thinking, you will set yourself up for success and will not fall off of your plan completely after one slip up.

Healthy Lifestyle Changes

One important way to ensure that these healthy choices stick for good is by changing some aspects of your lifestyle. By doing this, you will reduce the chances of slipping up by eliminating them altogether. For example, you can change the way you approach the grocery store.

When you are entering the grocery store, it is important that you change a few things about the way you shop, in order to set yourself up for success. This is especially important when you are just beginning your intuitive eating practice, as it will be challenging for you to enter the grocery store and avoid cravings and temptations.

The first thing to keep in mind when grocery shopping for a new diet is to enter with a list. By doing this, you are giving yourself a guide to follow, which will prevent you from picking up things that you are craving or things that you feel like eating in that moment.

One of the biggest things to keep in mind when beginning a new eating practice like intuitive eating is to avoid shopping when you are hungry. This will make you reach for anything and everything that you see. By entering the grocery store when you are satiated or when you have just eaten, you will be able to stick to your list and avoid falling prey to temptations.

If you treat your grocery shopping experience like a treasure hunt, you will be able to cross things off of the list one at a time without venturing to the parts of the grocery store that will prove to be a challenge for you to resist. If you are making healthy eating choices, you will likely be spending most of your time at the perimeter of the grocery store. This is where the whole, plant-based foods are located. By doing this, and entering with a list, you will be able to avoid the middle aisles where the processed, high-sugar temptation foods are all kept.

Having a plan is key when it comes to succeeding in learning new habits and employing a new lifestyle. This plan can be as detailed as you wish, or it can simply come in the form of a general overview. I recommend you start with a more detailed plan in the beginning as you ease into things.

As everyone is different, you may be the type of person who likes lots of lists and plans, or you may be the type of person who doesn't, but for everyone, beginning with a plan and following it closely for the first little while is best. For example, this plan can include things like what you will focus on each week, what you will reduce your intake of, and what you will try to achieve in terms of the mental work involved.

Once you have come up with a general plan for your new lifestyle and how you want it to look, you can then begin laying out more specific plans.

Planning your individual meals will make it much easier for you when you get home from work or when you wake up tired in the morning and need to pack something for your lunch.

You can plan your meals out a week in advance, two weeks or even a month if you wish. You can post this up on your fridge, and each day you will know exactly what you are eating, with no thinking required. This way, there won't be a chance for you to consider ordering a pizza or heating up some chicken fingers because you will already know exactly what you are going to make. By approaching your new style of eating in this way, you can make this transition easier on yourself and ensure success every step of the way.

30-Day Meal Plan

The following 30-day meal plan includes a variety of meals that you can make in order to keep your first thirty days interesting and tasty!

Day 1

- Breakfast:

Coffee

Feta, mushroom and spinach, omelet.

- Lunch:

Oven-baked tempeh with broccoli and cauliflower rice.

- Dinner:

Chicken Caesar salad- tofu and romaine lettuce, parmesan

Day 2

- Breakfast:

Unsweetened yogurt with a mix of some berries such as strawberries, raspberries, and some seeds like flax seeds and chia seeds, and nuts like sliced almonds and walnuts.

- Lunch:

A healthy lunch-time salad with avocado, cheese, grape tomatoes, and a variety of nuts and seeds like spicy pumpkin seeds. Add a salad dressing on top such as blue cheese or ranch dressing, or a homemade one using olive oil and garlic.

- Dinner:

Chicken breast with onions and a homemade tomato sauce. Served alongside some grilled zucchini or eggplant.

Day 3

- Breakfast:

A no sugar added full fat Greek yogurt bowl with seeds, nuts and berries.

1 Cup of coffee

- Lunch:

Make your own lunch box, including firm tofu or meat of some sort, raw tomatoes, any type of cheese cubes that you wish, pickles, a hard-boiled egg, vegetables such as celery, carrots, radishes or zucchini, nuts for protein and fat such as walnuts, or almonds, homemade guacamole (avocado, onion, garlic, jalapeno).

- Dinner:

Grilled portobello, grilled eggplant and grilled zucchini as well as cherry tomatoes sautéed in extra virgin olive oil with garlic. Served with rice and protein such as pork or chicken.

Day 4

- Breakfast:

Coffee

Homemade mushroom & Spinach Frittata, including any vegetables that you wish such as bell peppers and onion.

- Lunch:

Cream cheese with cucumber slices for dipping.

Hard-boiled egg

Meatballs with sweet and sour sauce

- Dinner

Bacon, Avocado, Lettuce, Tomato panini.

Day 5

- Breakfast:

Egg Salad with lettuce, cucumber and whole grain bread.

- Lunch:

Homemade guacamole (avocado, onion, garlic, jalapeno, lime juice) with raw zucchini slices for dipping.

Hard-boiled egg

Tuna

- Dinner:

Cauliflower gratin (cheese, cauliflower, onion, garlic and so on)

As well as chopped lettuce drizzled with Caesar Dressing

Day 6

- Breakfast:

Coffee with heavy cream or coconut oil.

Celery sticks, dipped in peanut or Almond Butter

- Lunch:

Leftover cauliflower gratin

As well as chopped lettuce drizzled with Caesar Dressing

- Dinner:

Cooked or raw broccoli with grated cheese on top

Steak seared in olive oil

Day 7

- Breakfast:

Pancakes with fresh fruits

Black Coffee

- Lunch:

Cold pasta salad with fresh vegetables

Feta and Tomato Meatballs

Raw fresh spinach

- Dinner:

Spicy Spaghetti Squash Casserole

Fresh spinach, raw or cooked with 1 Tbsp ranch dressing drizzled on top.

Day 8

- Breakfast

Smoothie

- Lunch

Tempeh meatballs with guacamole and raw vegetable salad

- Dinner

Rice noodle stir fry with your choice of vegetables and tofu

Day 9

- Breakfast

Omelet cooked in coconut oil with cheese, onions, bell pepper and tomatoes

- Lunch

Tofu scramble with vegetables such as spinach and mushrooms and cheese

- Dinner

Curry with chicken, rice and coconut milk sauce with hot chili paste

Day 10

- Breakfast

Full fat yogurt unsweetened with berries, chia seeds, flax seeds

- Lunch

Cobb salad with boiled egg, vegetables of your choice, tofu, tempeh or chicken and Caesar dressing

- Dinner

Homemade pizza with your choice of toppings

Day 11

- Breakfast

Smoothie with chia seeds and flax seeds, berries and plant-based protein powder, as well as plant-based milk

- Lunch

Salad with tofu or boiled egg, olive oil dressing, spinach and diced vegetables

- Dinner

Vegetarian frittata using coconut oil, spinach, mushroom, cheese, bell peppers and tomato

Day 12

- Breakfast

Greek yogurt no sugar added with nuts and seeds

- Lunch

Homemade tacos with your choice of toppings, including ground turkey

- Dinner

Macaroni and cheese with crumbled roasted bread crumbs on top

Day 13

- Breakfast

Whole grain oats with no sugar added, nuts, flax and chia seeds as well as heavy cream and a plant-based nut butter.

- Lunch

Lettuce wraps with curried tofu and grilled eggplant and zucchini

- Dinner

Homemade burritos filled with crumbled, seasoned meat of your choice, sour cream, guacamole and diced tomatoes

Day 14

- Breakfast

Greek yogurt no sugar added with nuts and seeds

- Lunch

Avocado egg bowls with bacon

- Dinner

Fried rice with your choice of vegetables, scrambled egg and tofu

Day 15

- Breakfast

Coffee with heavy cream and no sugar added

- Lunch

Carrots with guacamole, cottage cheese with nuts and seeds and homemade baked zucchini chips with olive oil drizzle

- Dinner

Egg Salad with Lettuce Wraps

Day 16

- Breakfast

Pancakes with no sugar added maple syrup

- Lunch

Vegetarian egg quiche with spinach and mushroom

- Dinner

Broccoli salad with onion, a cheese of your choice, creamy ranch dressing, almonds and walnuts sliced, as well as some avocado and tofu cubes

Day 17

- Breakfast

Potato hash browns fried in olive oil, sunny side up egg and tempeh "bacon" with a side of grilled tomatoes

- Lunch

Avocadoes stuffed with cauliflower "taco meat", homemade salsa with tomatoes and herbs, sour cream, and grated cheese

- Dinner

Cooked or raw broccoli

Small amount of butter that can be added to the broccoli for taste

Grated cheese on top that can also be added to the broccoli

With steak seared in olive oil

Day 18

- Breakfast

Shakshuka with eggs, tomatoes and parsley

- Lunch

Grilled zucchini roll ups with tomato and cheese

- Dinner

Coconut milk curry with rice, bell peppers and tofu

Day 19

- Breakfast

Breakfast smoothie with berries, no sugar added and full fat milk

- Lunch

Broccoli and cheese fritters with homemade hummus to dip and a side of carrots, celery and cucumber for dipping

- Dinner

Cobb salad including hard-boiled egg, ham cubes, your choice of vegetables and an olive oil or ranch dressing

Day 20

- Breakfast

Spinach and mushroom frittata

- Lunch

Sandwich with scrambled eggs, spinach and mushrooms cooked in olive oil and topped with lettuce, tomato or any other fillings or toppings you wish to include. Finally, add a homemade creamy avocado sauce with avocado, cilantro, pepper and salt and some sour cream.

- Dinner

Rice risotto with cheese, vegetable broth and mushrooms

Day 21

- Breakfast

Unsweetened yogurt with a mix of berries such as strawberries, raspberries, and some seeds like flax seeds and chia seeds, and nuts like sliced almonds and walnuts.

- Lunch

Caesar salad- dressing with no sugar added

Raw vegetables, mixed greens and tempeh

- Dinner

Cauliflower gratin- cheese, cauliflower and choice of vegetables

Day 22

- Breakfast

Hash browns fried in olive oil, sunny side up egg and bacon with a side of grilled tomatoes

- Lunch

Stuffed half zucchini with feta cheese, tomato sauce (no sugar added) and herbs for topping

- Dinner

Mashed potatoes using whole milk and cheese, with grilled eggplant and mushrooms

Day 23

- Breakfast

Nut butter smoothie with yogurt, nut butter, flax seeds, chia seeds

- Lunch

Pan fried steak seasoned with herbs and olive oil, paired with

A spinach salad with raw vegetables of choice and no sugar added Caesar dressing

- Dinner

Cauliflower pasta salad with celery, spinach, onions, and walnuts

Day 24

- Breakfast

Feta, mushroom and Spinach, omelet

Coffee

- Lunch

Coleslaw with a creamy cilantro dressing, carrots, cabbage, celery, tomato and herbs for topping

- Dinner

Crispy tofu cubes with zucchini noodles and a homemade peanut sauce

Day 25

- Breakfast

No bake protein bars

Coffee with no sugar added

- Lunch

Roasted tomatoes with goat cheese, spinach, cilantro and olive oil & balsamic drizzle

- Dinner

Eggplant and zucchini "French fries" with olive oil and crispy tofu cubes

Baked chicken breast

Day 26

- Breakfast

Pancakes with no sugar added maple syrup, full fat Greek yogurt and berries for topping

- Lunch

Low carb broccoli cheese soup with crispy cauliflower on the side

- Dinner

Curried rice with choice of vegetables, such as bell peppers and broccoli

Day 27

- Breakfast

Breakfast salad with scrambled egg, avocado, mixed greens, grilled tomatoes and cheese

- Lunch

Fried goat cheese with roasted red peppers, spinach and olive oil drizzle

- Dinner

Spicy Spaghetti Squash Casserole

Fresh spinach, raw or cooked with ranch dressing drizzled on top

Day 28

- Breakfast

Full fat yogurt unsweetened with berries, chia seeds, flax seeds

- Lunch

Vegetarian chili with tomato, sour cream, a variety of beans and tomatoes

- Dinner

Zucchini spiral pasta noodles with creamy yogurt avocado sauce

Day 29

- Breakfast

Cauliflower "bread" grilled cheese sandwich (similar to cauliflower crust pizza but made as a grilled cheese sandwich instead.

- Lunch

Green beans with mushrooms and tomatoes with a chicken breast on the side

- Dinner

Grape tomato marinara on pasta noodles with parmigiano Reggiano cheese and fresh cracked pepper.

Day 30

- Breakfast

Egg taco shells filled with choice of vegetables

- Lunch

Baked crispy tofu steaks with a sesame seed crust on a bed of zucchini strips and spinach

- Dinner

Baked Spaghetti squash filled with roasted tomatoes and eggplant, topped with melted, crispy cheese

Chapter 7: What to Do Next

As you take all of this information forth with you, it may seem overwhelming to begin applying this to your own life. Remember, life is a process, and you do not need to expect perfection from yourself right away. By taking the first step-reading this book, you are already on your way to changing your life. If you fall off and find that you are back to your old ways, try to find inspiration in the pages of this book once again. If you find that you are unable to find success on your own, there is no shame in seeking professional help. There are many people who are trained professionals in dealing with disordered eating and who can serve as a mentor or a guide for you as you navigate this challenge.

How To Seek Help If It Becomes Uncontrollable?

Understanding and accepting that you need help is the first step to recovery. By reading this book, you have taken this step. If you need further help, there is no shame in accepting this fact. There are many ways to seek help for disordered eating, depending on the level of help that you need. Below is a list of ways that you can seek help, ordered from least to most help.

- Online resources
- Support System
- Support Group
- Group counseling
- Anonymous online counseling or telephone counseling
- One on One counseling

- Talk therapy
- Rehab centers

Counseling or Therapy

Talking therapies are very effective treatments for disordered eating. The things that people learn in therapy gives them the insight and skills in order to feel better and tackle their eating disorder, as well as to prevent it from coming back in the future.

One example of talk therapy is Cognitive Behavioral Therapy or CBT. The way that cognitive behavioral therapy works is by putting an emphasis on the relationship between a person's thoughts, emotions, and behaviors. The theory behind this is that when a person changes any one of these components, change will be initiated in the others. The goal of CBT is to help a person decrease negative thoughts or the amount of worry they experience in order to increase their overall quality of life.

If you think that this is something you would benefit from, please reach out to your local resources to find out more.

PART II

Are you worried that your hormones are not at their optimal levels? Here is a diet that will solve your problems.

Chapter 1: Health Benefits of the Hormone Diet

When it comes to getting healthy through weight loss, there's never any shortage of fitness crazes and diets that claim to have the secret to easy and sustainable weight loss. One of the latest diet plans that have come into the spotlight is the hormone diet, which claims that people often struggle to lose weight because of their hormones.

A hormone diet is a 3-step process that spans over six weeks and is designed to synchronize your hormones and promote a healthy body through detoxification, nutritional supplements, exercise, and diet. The diet controls what you eat and informs you about the correct time to eat to ensure maximum benefits to your hormones. Many books have been written on this topic with supporters of the diet assuring people that they can lose weight quickly and significantly through diet and exercise and reset or manipulate their hormones. Although the diet has a few variations, the central idea around each is that correcting the body's perceived hormonal imbalances is the key to losing weight.

The most important benefit of a hormone diet is that it takes a solid stance on improving overall health through weight loss and promoting regular exercise as well as natural, nutritious foods. Apart from that, it also focuses on adequate sleep, stress management, emotional health, and other healthy lifestyle habits that are all essential components that people should follow, whether it's a part of a diet or not. Including a water diet, it aims towards losing about twelve pounds in the 1st phase and 2 pounds a week after that.

Hormones have an essential role in the body's everyday processes, like helping bones grow, digesting food, etc. They act as "chemical messengers," instructing the cells to perform specific actions and are transported around the body through the bloodstream.

One of the very important food items to be included in the hormone diet is salmon. Salmon is rich in omega-3 fatty acids, Docosahexaenoic acid, and Eicosapentaenoic acid (EPA). It is rich in selenium too. These help to lower your blood pressure and also reduce the level of unhealthy cholesterol in the blood. These make you less prone to heart diseases. Salmon is a rich source of healthy fat. If consumed in sufficient amounts, it provides you energy and helps you get rid of unwanted body fat. Salmon is well-known for giving fantastic weight loss results as it has less saturated fat, unlike other protein sources. Salmon is packed with vitamins like vitamin-k, E, D, and A. These are extremely helpful for your eyes, bone joints, etc. These vitamins are also good for your brain, regulation of metabolic balance, and repairing your muscles. Salmon's vitamins and omega-3 fatty acids are amazing for sharpening your mind. It also improves your memory retention power. If you consume salmon, you are less likely to develop dementia or mental dis-functions. Salmon has anti-inflammatory properties and is low in omega-6 fatty acid content (which is pro-inflammatory in nature and is present in a huge amount in the modern diet). It promotes healthy skin and gives you radiant and glowing skin. It is good for the winter because it helps you to stay warm. It also provides lubrication to your joints because of the abundant presence of essential minerals and fatty acids in it. Apart from this, some other things to include in your diet are arugula, kale, ginger, avocado, carrots, and so on.

There are almost sixteen hormones that can influence weight. For example, the hormone leptin produced by your fat cells is considered a "satiety hormone," which makes you feel full by reducing your appetite. As a signaling hormone, it communicates with the part of your brain (hypothalamus) that controls food intake and appetite. Leptin informs the brain when there is enough fat in storage, and extra fat is not required. This helps prevent overeating. Individuals who are obese or overweight generally have very high levels of leptin in their blood. Research shows that the level of leptin in obese individuals was almost four times higher than that in individuals with normal weight.

Studies have found that fat hormones like leptin and adiponectin can promote long-term weight loss by reducing appetite and increasing metabolism. It is believed that both these fat hormones follow the same pathway in the brain to manage blood sugar (glucose) and body weight (Robert V. Considine, 1996).

Simply put, the hormone diet works by helping to create a calorie deficit through better nutritional habits and exercise, which ultimately results in weight loss. It's also essential to consult a doctor before following this detox diet or consuming any dietary supplements.

Chapter 2: Hormone-Rebalancing Smoothies

Estrogen Detox Smoothie

Total Prep & Cooking Time: 5 minutes

Yields: One glass

Nutrition Facts: Calories: 312 | Carbs: 47.9g | Protein: 18.6g | Fat: 8.5g | Fiber: 3g

Ingredients:

- Half a cup of hemp seeds
- Two kiwis (medium-sized)
- A quarter each of
  - Avocado (medium-sized)
  - Cucumber (medium-sized)
- Half a unit each of
  - Lemon (squeezed freshly)
  - Green apple
- One celery (medium-sized)
- A quarter cup of cilantro
- Two tbsps. of chis seeds
- Two cups of water (filtered)
- One tsp. of cacao nibs

- One tbsp. of coconut oil

Method:

1. Blend the ingredients all together to form a smoothie at high speed. The thickness can be adjusted according to your preference by adding more water to the mixture.

2. Serve and enjoy.

Dopamine Delight Smoothie

Total Prep Time: 10 minutes

Yields: One serving

Nutrition Facts: Calories: 383 | Carbs: 31g | Protein: 24g | Fat: 18.g | Fiber: 3g

Ingredients:

- Half a teaspoon of cinnamon (ground)
- Half a cup of peeled banana (the bananas must be frozen)
- One organic espresso, double shot (measuring half a cup)
- One tablespoon of chia seeds
- A three-fourth cup of soy milk (plain or vanilla-flavored)
- Protein powder, a serving (from the whey with the flavor of vanilla)

Method:

1. Fill in the bowl of your blender with all the ingredients (from the section of ingredients) except the whey protein powder and then proceed by switching to a high-speed blending option. Make sure it acquires a smooth consistency and then pour it out.

2. Now you may add the protein powder and give it another shot of blend until the whole things get incorporated, a bit of the goat cheese (already crumbled).

Breakfast Smoothie Bowl

Total Prep Time: 10 minutes

Yields: 2 servings

Nutrition Facts: Calories: 290 | Carbs: 53g | Protein: 6g | Fat: 8g | Fiber: 9g

Ingredients:

- One cup of thoroughly rinsed blueberries (fresh and ripe)
- A sundry of nuts and fruits for garnishing, which includes – strawberries, bananas (thinly sliced), peanuts (Spanish), kiwi (chopped), segments of tangerine, and raspberries.
- One cup of Greek yogurt

For the preparation of honey flax granola,

- Two tablespoons each of
  o Flaxseeds
  o Vegetable oil
- Oats (old-fashioned), approximately a cup
- One tablespoon of honey

Method:

1. Set your oven at a temperature of 350 degrees F.

2. Preparation of the smoothie: collect the diverse types of berries, wash them thoroughly, and then put them in the blender and turn it on. Make an even mixture out of it. Add some amount of the yogurt and blend it again to form a smooth texture.

3. For preparing the granola: Take a small-sized bowl and then drizzle a few drops oil in it. Then add the oats, flax, and honey to the oil, one by one, and mix it well. You are required to toss the bowl thoroughly to get the mixture well-coated with the poured oil. After you are done, place the oats mixture in a baking sheet evenly. Bake it for about twenty minutes. This mark will be enough to give the oats a beautiful tinge of golden brown. Allow it to cool.

4. Now you will require a shallow bowl to spoon in some yogurt, and this will be the first layer. Form a second layer with the various fruits and nuts and finally for the third layer, top with the granola.

5. Enjoy.

Notes:

- *Using frozen nuts and fruits in a warm-weather will get much to your relief.*

- *For a vegan smoothie bowl, sub the yogurt with coconut or almond yogurt.*

- *Give the pan a few strokes while baking the oats.*

Blueberry Detox Smoothie

Total Prep Time: Ten minutes

Yields: One serving

Nutrition Facts: Calories: 326 | Carbs: 65g | Protein: 4g | Fat: 8g | Fiber: 9g

Ingredients:

- One cup of wild blueberries (frozen)
- One banana (sliced into several pieces) frozen
- Orange juice (approximately half a cup)
- Cilantro leaves, fresh (approximately a measuring a small handful size)
- A quarter of an entire avocado
- A quarter cup of water

Method:

1. Add cilantro, avocado, water, blueberries, banana, and orange juice in the blender and then process.

2. Make the ingredients integrated so well that they become smooth in their consistency.

Notes: *It is recommended that you add the potent herb, cilantro, or parsley in a small amount when consuming this smoothie for the first time, as it might trigger a mild headache. If you do* *not get a headache, you may add a bit more of the cilantro leaves.*

Maca Mango Smoothie

Total Prep & Cooking Time: 2 minutes

Yields: 2 servings

Nutrition Facts: Calories: 53 | Carbs: 13g | Protein: 1g | Fat: 3g | Fiber: 1.5g

Ingredients:

- One and a half cups each of
  - Fresh mango
  - Frozen mango
- One tablespoon each of
  - Ground flaxseed
  - Nut butter
- One teaspoon of ground turmeric
- Two teaspoons of maca root powder
- Three-quarter cups of nut milk
- One frozen banana

Method:

1. Blend all the ingredients together to get a smooth mixture.

2. Adjust consistency by adding nut milk.

3. Once done, divide into two glasses and enjoy!

Pituitary Relief Smoothie

Total Prep & Cooking Time: 5 minutes

Yields: 2 servings

Nutrition Facts: Calories: 174 | Carbs: 18.3g | Protein: 9.7g | Fat: 8.3g | Fiber: 14.4g

Ingredients:

- One teaspoon of coconut oil
- One fresh or frozen ripe banana
- One tablespoon of raw sesame seeds
- Two teaspoons each of
  - Chia seeds
  - Raw Maca powder
  - Raw Spirulina
- Two cups of water
- Two tablespoons of hulled hemp seeds

Method:

1. You have to use a blender to process this smoothie. Add the hulled hemp seeds, sesame seeds, and water in the blender and process them. Do it at

high speed, and it will only require a minute. This will give you raw-milk like texture.

2. Then, add the following ingredients into it – coconut oil, banana, chia seeds, Maca, and Spirulina, and process the ingredients once again but this time on medium speed for another minute or so. Everything will become well incorporated.

3. You have to drink this smoothie on an empty stomach.

Notes: *In order to make the smoothie rich in antioxidants, you can add some fresh fruits like blueberries, kiwi, and raspberries.*

Chapter 2: Easy Breakfast Recipes

Scrambled Eggs With Feta and Tomatoes

Total Prep & Cooking Time: 10 minutes

Yields: One Plate

Nutrition Facts: Calories: 421 | Carbs: 8.6g | Protein: 20.3g | Fat: 35.1g | Fiber: 1.6g

Ingredients:

- One tbsp. each of
  - Olive oil (extra virgin)
  - Freshly chopped parsley, basil, dill or chives
- Half a cup of cherry tomatoes (each tomato sliced into half)
- Two ounces of crumbled feta cheese (approximately a quarter cup)
- Two eggs are beaten
- Two tbsp. of onion (diced)
- To taste:
  - Black pepper
  - Kosher salt

Method:

1. Keep the beaten eggs in a small-sized bowl and then season it with a pinch of pepper and salt. Set the bowl aside.

2. Use a nonstick skillet to proceed with the cooking. Pour two tbsp. of olive oil. Then add the diced onions. Stir over moderate heat and cook until softened. Make sure that the onions do not look brown. This process should get done by a minute.

3. Add half a cup of tomatoes to skillet and then continue to mix for about two minutes.

4. Now you may add the eggs. Using a spatula, gather the beaten eggs to the center by moving spatula all over the skillet.

5. The eggs will take an additional minute to get cooked. So after that mark, add the parsley or other herbs (if preferred) and feta cheese. Keep the eggs underdone as they will get cooked completely after they are served in the plate itself (from the residual heat). Therefore, cook the entire thing in the skillet for 30 seconds only.

6. Take a serving plate and transfer the eggs to it. Top with some sprinkled parsley and feta cheese, drizzled with some oil, and seasoned with some pepper and salt. These additions are optional and may vary as per your desire.

Smashed Avo and Quinoa

Total Prep & Cooking Time: 15 minutes

Yields: Six bowls

Nutrition Facts: Calories: 492 | Carbs: 67g | Protein: 15g | Fat: 20g | Fiber: 13g

Ingredients:

- One avocado skinned, cut into half, and then pitted
- A handful of cilantro or coriander
- Half a lemon (juiced)
- A quarter red onion (diced finely)
- One-eighth teaspoon of cayenne pepper
- To taste: Sea salt

For the Greens,

- One handful of kale
- One handful of soft herbs (basil, parsley or mint)
- One handful of chard or spinach
- For frying: butter or coconut oil

Serve with,

- One cup of quinoa (cooked)

Method:

1. You will require a frying pan to get this done. To it, add the coconut oil or butter (whichever you prefer) and add the greens. Toss them carefully and then sauté over moderate heat. Stop when they become soft.

2. Mix the onion, cayenne, avocado, cilantro, salt, lemon, and pepper to a bowl and mix them completely. The pepper and salt must be added according to the taste.

3. Add cooked quinoa to the tossed greens and heat altogether over low heat.

4. Take a serving plate and place the quinoa mixture and greens to it. Crown the whole thing with smashed avocado and then serve.

Hormone Balancing Granola

Total Prep & Cooking Time: 35 minutes

Yields: 8 servings

Nutrition Facts: Calories: 360 | Carbs: 19.8g | Protein: 5.1g | Fat: 28.8g | Fiber: 5.8g

Ingredients:

- One-third cup each of
  - Flaxseed meal
  - Pumpkin seeds
  - Seedless raisins
- Two teaspoons of cinnamon
- One teaspoon of vanilla extract
- Four tablespoons of maple syrup
- Five tablespoons of melted coconut oil
- A quarter cup of unsweetened coconut flakes
- Two-thirds cup each of
  - Chopped pecans
  - Chopped brazil nuts
- Two tablespoons of ground chia seeds

Method:

1. Set the temperature of the oven to 180 degrees F and preheat.

2. In a food processor, chop the pecans and the Brazil nuts. Then, mix these chopped nuts with coconut flakes, seeds, and other nuts present in the list of ingredients.

3. Add maple syrup, coconut oil, cinnamon, and vanilla extract in a separate bowl and combine well.

4. Now, take the wet ingredients and pour them into the dry ingredients. Mix thoroughly so that everything has become coated properly.

5. Place the prepared mixture in the oven for half an hour and cook.

6. Once done, cut into pieces and serve.

Chapter 3: Healthy Lunch Recipes

Easy Shakshuka

Total Prep & Cooking Time: 30 minutes

Yields: Six servings

Nutrition Facts: Calories: 154 | Carbs: 4.1g | Protein: 9g | Fat: 7.8g | Fiber: 0g

Ingredients:

- Olive oil (extra virgin)
- Two chopped green peppers
- One teaspoon each of
  - Paprika (sweet)
  - Coriander (ground)
- A pinch of red pepper (flakes)
- Half a cup of tomato sauce
- A quarter cup each of
  - Mint leaves (freshly chopped)
  - Parsley leaves (chopped freshly)
- One yellow onion, large-sized (chopped)
- Two cloves of garlic, chopped
- Half a teaspoon of cumin (ground)
- Six cups of chopped tomatoes (Vine-ripe)

- Six large-sized eggs
- To taste: Pepper and salt

Method:

1. You will require a large-sized skillet (made of cast iron). Pour three tablespoons of oil and heat it. After bringing the oil to boil, add the peppers, spices, onions, garlic, pepper, and salt. Stir time to time to cook the veggies for five minutes until they become softened.

2. After the vegetables become soft, add the chopped tomatoes and then tomato sauce. Cover the skillet and simmer for an additional fifteen minutes.

3. Now, you may remove the lid from the pan and then cook a touch more to thicken the consistency. At this point, you may adjust the taste.

4. Make six cavities within the tomato mixture and crack one egg each inside the cavities.

5. Cover the skillet after reducing the heat and allow it to cook so that the eggs settle into the cavities.

6. Keep track of the time and accordingly uncover the skillet and then add mint and parsley. Season with more black and red pepper according to your desire. Serve them warm with the sort of bread you wish.

Ginger Chicken

Total Prep & Cooking Time: 50 minutes

Yields: Six Servings

Nutrition Facts: Calories: 310 | Carbs: 6g | Protein: 37g | Fat: 16g | Fiber: 1g

Ingredients:

- A one-kilogram pack of chicken thighs (skinless and boneless)
- Four cloves of garlic (chopped finely)
- A fifteen-gram pack of coriander (fresh and chopped)
- Two tablespoons of sunflower oil
- One teaspoon each of
  o Turmeric (ground)
  o Chili powder (mild)
- A four hundred milliliter can of coconut milk (reduced-fat)
- One cube of chicken stock
- One ginger properly peeled and chopped finely (it should be of the size of a thumb)
- One lime, juiced
- Two medium-sized onions
- One red chili, sliced and the seeds removed (fresh)

Method:

1. Make the chicken thighs into three large chunks and marinate them with chili powder, garlic, coriander (half of the entire amount), ginger, oil (one tbsp.), and lime juice. Cover the bowl after stirring them well and then store it in the fridge until oven-ready.

2. Marinade the chicken and keep overnight for better flavor.

3. Chop the onions finely (it is going to be the simplest for preparing the curry) before dropping them into the food processor. Pour oil into the frying pan (large-sized) and heat it. Then add chopped onions and stir them thoroughly for eight minutes until the pieces become soft. Then pour the turmeric powder and stir for an additional minute.

4. Now add the chicken mixture and cook on high heat until you notice a change in its color. Pour the chicken stock, chili, and coconut milk and after covering the pan simmer for another twenty minutes. Sprinkle the left-over coriander leaves and then serve hot.

5. Enjoy.

Carrot and Miso Soup

Total Prep & Cooking Time: 1 hour

Yields: Four bowls of soup

Nutrition Facts: Calories: 76 | Carbs: 8.76g | Protein: 4.83g | Fat: 2.44g | Fiber: 1.5g

Ingredients:

- Two tbsps. of oil
- Garlic, minced (four cloves)
- One inch of garlic (grated)
- Three tbsps. of miso paste (white)
- One diced onion
- One pound of carrot (sliced thinly)
- Four cups of vegetable stock
- To taste: Pepper and Salt

For garnishing,

- Two scallions (sliced thinly)
- Chili pepper (seven spices)
- One nori roasted (make thin slivers)
- Sesame oil

Method:

1. Using a soup pot will be convenient to proceed with. Pour oil in a pot and then heat over a high flame. Now you may put garlic, carrot, and onion and sauté them thoroughly. Cook for about ten minutes so that the onions turn translucent.

2. Then add the ginger and vegetable stock. Mix them well and cook all together. Put the flame to simmer. Cover the pot while cooking to make the carrot tender. This will take another thirty minutes.

3. Put off the flame and puree the soup with the help of an immersion blender.

4. Use a small-sized bowl to whisk together a spoonful of the soup and the white miso paste. Stir until the paste dissolve and pour the mixture back to the pot.

5. Add pepper and salt if required.

6. Divide the soup among four bowls and enrich its feel by adding scallions, sesame oil, seven spices, and nori.

Arugula Salad

Total Prep & Cooking Time: 1 hour 10 minutes

Yields: Two bowls of salad

Nutrition Facts: Calories: 336.8 | Carbs: 30.6g | Protein: 7.7g | Fat: 22.2g | Fiber: 7.3g

Ingredients:

For the salad,

- Two medium-sized beets (boiled or roasted for about an hour), skinned and sliced into pieces that can easily be bitten
- Four tablespoons of goat cheese
- Approximately 2.5 oz. of baby arugula (fresh)
- A quarter cup of walnuts (chopped roughly before toasting)

For the dressing,

- Three tablespoons of olive oil (extra virgin)
- A quarter tsp. each of
  - Mustard powder (dried)
  - Pepper
- Half a tsp. each of
  - Salt
  - Sugar

- One and a half tablespoons of lemon juice

Method:

1. For preparing the vinaigrette, place all the ingredients (listed in the dressing ingredients section) in a jar and then shake them to emulsify. At this stage, before starting with the process of emulsification, you may add or remove the ingredients as per your liking.

2. Get the salad assembled (again depending upon the taste you want to give it), add a fistful of arugula leaves, place some chopped beets (after they have been cooked), and finally the toasted walnuts (already chopped).

3. Drizzle vinaigrette over the salad and enjoy.

Notes:

- *Coat the beets with oil (olive), roll them up in an aluminum foil, and then roast the beets at a temperature of 400 degrees F.*

- *And for boiling the beets, immerse them in water after transferring to a pot and simmer them for 45 minutes.*

Kale Soup

Total Prep & Cooking Time: 55 minutes

Yields: 8 servings

Nutrition Facts: Calories: 277.3 | Carbs: 50.9g | Protein: 9.6g | Fat: 4.5g | Fiber: 10.3g

Ingredients:

- Two tbsps. of dried parsley
- One tbsp. of Italian seasoning
- Salt and pepper
- Thirty oz. of drained cannellini beans
- Six peeled and cubed white potatoes
- Fifteen ounces of diced tomatoes
- Six vegetable Bouillon cubes
- Eight cups of water
- One bunch of kale (with chopped leaves and stems removed)
- Two tbsps. of chopped garlic
- One chopped yellow onion
- Two tbsps. of olive oil

Method:

1. At first, take a large soup pot, add in some olive oil, and heat it.

2. Add garlic and onion. Cook them until soft.

3. Then stir in the kale and cook for about two minutes, until wilted.

4. Pour the water and add the beans, potatoes, tomatoes, vegetable bouillon, parsley, and the Italian seasoning.

5. On medium heat, simmer the soup for about twenty-five minutes, until the potatoes are cooked through.

6. Finally, do the seasoning with salt and pepper according to your taste.

Roasted Sardines

Total Prep & Cooking Time: 25 minutes

Yields: 4 servings

Nutrition Facts: Calories: 418 | Carbs: 2.6g | Protein: 41g | Fat: 27.2g | Fiber: 0.8g

Ingredients:

- 3.5 oz. of cherry tomatoes (cut them in halves)
- One medium-sized red onion (chopped finely)
- Two tablespoons each of
  - Chopped parsley
  - Extra-virgin olive oil
- One clove of garlic (halved)
- Eight units of fresh sardines (gutted and cleaned, heads should be cleaned)
- A quarter teaspoon of chili flakes
- One teaspoon of toasted cumin seeds
- Half a lemon (zested and juiced)

Method:

1. Set the temperature of the oven to 180 degrees C and preheat. Take a roasting tray and grease it lightly.

2. Take a bowl and add the tomatoes and onions in it. Add the lemon juice too and toss the veggies in the lemon juice. Now, add the zest, olive oil, chili, cumin, garlic, and parsley and toss everything once again.

3. Use pepper and salt to season the mixture. The cavity of the sardines has to be filled. Use some of the tomato and onion mixture for this purpose. Once done, place the sardines on the prepared roasting tray. Take the remaining mixture and scatter it over the sardines.

4. Roast the sardines for about 10-15 minutes, and by the end of this, they should be cooked thoroughly.

5. Serve and enjoy!

Chapter 4: Tasty Dinner Recipes

Corned Beef and Cabbage

Total Prep & Cooking Time: 2 hours 35 minutes

Yields: 5 servings

Nutrition Facts: Calories: 868.8 | Carbs: 75.8g | Protein: 50.2g | Fat: 41.5g |
Fiber: 14g

Ingredients:

- One big cabbage head (cut it into small wedges)
- Five peeled carrots (chopped into three-inch pieces)
- Ten red potatoes (small)
- Three pounds of corned beef brisket (along with the packet of spice)

Method:

1. At first, in a Dutch oven or a large pot, place the corned beef, and cover
   it with water. Then add in the spices from the packet of spices that came
   along with the beef. Cover the pot, bring it to a boil, and finally reduce it
   to a simmer. Allow it to simmer for about 2 hours and 30 minutes or
   until tender.

2. Add carrots and whole potatoes, and cook them until the vegetables are tender. Add the cabbage wedges and cook for another fifteen minutes. Then finally remove the meat and allow it to rest for fifteen minutes.

3. Take a bowl, place the vegetables in it, and cover it. Add broth (which is reserved in the pot) as much as you want. Then finally cut the meat against the grain.

Rosemary Chicken

Total Prep & Cooking Time: 50 minutes

Yields: 4 servings

Nutrition Facts: Calories: 232 | Carbs: 3.9g | Protein: 26.7g | Fat: 11.6g | Fiber: 0.3g

Ingredients:

- Four chicken breast halves (skinless and boneless)
- One-eighth tsp. kosher salt
- One-fourth tsp. ground black pepper
- One and a half tbsps. of lemon juice
- One and a half tbsps. of Dijon mustard
- Two tbsps. of freshly minced rosemary
- Three tbsps. of olive oil
- Eight minced garlic cloves

Method:

1. At first, preheat a grill to medium-high heat. The grate needs to be lightly oiled.

2. Take a bowl and add lemon juice, mustard, rosemary, olive oil, garlic, salt, and ground black pepper. Whisk them together.

3. Take a resealable plastic bag and place the chicken breasts in it. Over the chicken, pour the garlic mixture (reserve one-eighth cup of it).

4. Seal the bag and start massaging the marinade gently into the chicken. Allow it to stand for about thirty minutes at room temperature.

5. Then on the preheated grill, place the chicken and cook for about four minutes.

6. Flip the chicken and baste it with the marinade reserved and then cook for about five minutes, until thoroughly cooked.

7. Finally, cover it with a foil and allow it to rest for about 2 minutes before you serve them.

Roasted Parsnips and Carrots

Total Prep & Cooking Time: 1 hour

Yields: 4 servings

Nutrition Facts: Calories: 112 | Carbs: 27g | Protein: 2g | Fat: 1g | Fiber: 7g

Ingredients:

- Two tbsps. of freshly minced parsley or dill
- One and a half tsp. of freshly ground black pepper
- One tbsp. kosher salt
- Three tbsps. of olive oil
- One pound of unpeeled carrots
- Two pounds of peeled parsnips

Method:

1. At first, preheat your oven to 425 degrees.

2. If the carrots and parsnips are thick, then cut them into halves lengthwise.

3. Then, slice each of them diagonally into one inch thick slices. Don't cut them too small because the vegetables will anyway shrink while you cook them.

4. Take a sheet pan, and place the cut vegetables on it.

5. Then add some olive oil, pepper, salt, and toss them nicely.

6. Roast them for about twenty to forty minutes (the roasting time depends on the size of the vegetables), accompanied by occasional tossing. Continue to roast until the carrots and parsnips become tender.

7. Finally, sprinkle some dill and serve.

Herbed Salmon

Total Prep & Cooking Time: 30 minutes

Yields: 4 servings

Nutrition Facts: Calories: 301 | Carbs: 1g | Protein: 29g | Fat: 19g | Fiber: 0g

Ingredients:

- Half a tsp. of dried thyme or two tsps. of freshly minced thyme
- Half a tsp. of pepper
- Three-fourth tsp. of salt
- One tbsp. of olive oil
- One tbsp. freshly minced rosemary or one tsp. of crushed dried rosemary.
- Four minced cloves of garlic
- Four (six ounces) fillets of salmon

Method:

1. At first, preheat your oven to 425 degrees.

2. Take a 15 by 10 by 1 inch baking pan and grease it.

3. Place the salmon on it while keeping the skin side down.

4. Combine the garlic cloves, rosemary, thyme, salt, and pepper. Spread it evenly over the salmon fillets.

5. Roast them for about fifteen to eighteen minutes until they reach your desired doneness.

Chipotle Cauliflower Tacos

Total Prep & Cooking Time: 30 minutes

Yields: 8 servings

Nutrition Facts: Calories: 440 | Carbs: 51.6g | Protein: 10.1g | Fat: 24g | Fiber: 9g

Ingredients:

For the tacos,

- Four tablespoons of avocado oil
- One head of cauliflower (large-sized, chopped into bite-sized florets)
- One cup of cilantro (freshly chopped)
- One tablespoon each of
    - Fresh lime juice
    - Maple syrup or honey
- Two tsps. of chipotle adobo sauce
- Cracked black pepper
- One teaspoon of salt
- 4-8 units of garlic cloves (freshly minced)

For the Chipotle Aioli,

- A quarter cup of chipotle adobo sauce
- Half a cup each of

- o   Sour cream
- o   Clean mayo

One teaspoon of sea salt

Two cloves of garlic (minced)

For serving,

- Almond flour tortillas
- Guacamole
- Almond ricotta cheese
- Sliced tomatoes, radish, and cabbage

Method:

1.   Set the temperature of the oven to 425 degrees F. Now, use parchment paper to line a pan. Take the bite-sized florets of the cauliflower and spread them evenly on the pan. Use 2-4 tbsps. of avocado oil, pepper, salt, and minced garlic and drizzle it on the pan.

2.   Roast the cauliflower for half an hour at 425 degrees F and halfway through the process, flip the florets.

3. When you are roasting the cauliflower, take the rest of the ingredients of the cauliflower and mix them in a bowl. Once everything has been properly incorporated, set the mixture aside.

4. Now, take another bowl and in it, add the ingredients of the chipotle aioli. Mix them and set the bowl aside.

5. If you have any other taco fixings, get them ready.

6. Once the cauliflower is ready, toss the florets in the chipotle sauce.

7. Serve the cauliflower in tortillas along with fixings of your choice and the chipotle aioli.

PART III

Chapter 1: Self-Confidence In Various Situations

"Each time we face our fear, we gain strength, courage, and confidence in the doing."

-Theodore Roosevelt

While we have been speaking of self-worth and self-value, the focus of this chapter will be self-confidence, which is a different subject altogether.

Self-confidence is when you have faith in yourself and your abilities in a particular situation, and it does not relate to overall self-worth. If your self-confidence levels are low, it is because you are not comfortable in a particular setting, for whatever reason.

To help make self-confidence more clear, here are a few scenarios that showcase it in different circumstances.

- A doctor is self-confident when he performs any type of procedure within his specialty. He has so much training and experience that he truly believes in his skills and abilities to perform in various situations at work. When this same doctor goes for a hike, he does not have the same level of confidence in conquering a high peak, because he is out of shape.

- A mechanic can fix any car with his eyes closed. He has been a mechanic for so many years, that he is confident there is nothing that will come into his garage that he cannot handle. When this mechanic tries to work on the plumbing in his home, he is not very successful and has no confidence in his ability to perform the tasks.

- A great artist is confident in his ability to paint a portrait. If you ask him to solve a math problem, he has no confidence whatsoever.

These examples showcase how self-confidence can truly be based on the state of affairs, depending on what a person is facing at the moment. To handle a situation well, you must have self-confidence in your ability to do so. Self-confidence is gained through training, education, repetition, and life experience. It is impossible to be confident in every situation you ever come across, but the more you are willing to learn, the more confidence you will gain throughout life.

How a Lack of Self-Confidence Affects Us

As I mentioned before, self-confidence is circumstantial and will impact various areas of your life differently. Depending on how much experience, knowledge, or training, we have in different aspects of life, our confidence will ebb and flow. The key is to have self-confidence in the important areas of our lives, where it really matters. There are many examples in our everyday lives where self-confidence will play a major role.

Regarding the work setting, people who lack confidence in this arena cannot perform their necessary duties at an adequate level. This means poor job performance, being overlooked for raises and promotions, and even being let go from a position. If a person performs their job well, low self-confidence can still impact their desire to move up the latter. If they are confident in their particular position but do not feel confident at a higher level, like management, then they won't go after the promotion. They will simply stay put, even though they have the potential to do more.

Concerning starting a business, a certain level of confidence is needed to perform numerous tasks. There are many independent skills involved in running a business, and chances are, you will be doing most of them yourself when you first start. You need to have the proper training and education in these different areas, like finance, setting a budget, and marketing, etc., or you will not succeed in them. If you feel you can't do them yourself, then you may have to higher someone to do so. It may be worth it to avoid errors.

Self-confidence matters in our personal lives too. In order to find friends or develop relationships, we must have confidence in our abilities to form them. For example, it takes a lot of confidence for a man to walk up to a woman and say, "hi." To make friends, you must have the courage to talk to people. To learn new things and experience a new adventure, you must also have confidence in yourself to perform them. Once again, confidence comes from experience, and the more you put yourself out there, the more confident you will become.

Confidence is crucial in specific social settings. For example, during a work meeting, a lack of confidence can hold you back from speaking up, even if you have something very important to say. You won't get the necessary information out there that many people in the meeting could receive value from. This also relates to socializing with friends. You may have a friend who is harming themselves, but because you are uncertain how they will react, you ca nothing. You do not have the confidence that you will be able to respond appropriately.

A lack of confidence does not allow you to communicate assertively, which is important in order to get what you want. Instead of asking for things directly, you will beat around the bush and hope that the person will pick up on your clues. You will also use minimizing language, like "Sort of" or "kind of." This type of communication makes it seem like you lack conviction, and no one will take you seriously. You will just appear weak. Being assertive is essential, whether you are asking for something at working or setting boundaries with your friends.

If you suffer from low self-confidence, then every aspect of your life will suffer. We will get into different ways of increasing your confidence in the next chapter. For now, we will discuss how self-confidence works in different settings, especially in those that create anxiety for everybody.

Chapter 2: Social Anxiety

For this chapter, I will provide more detail for a specific type of confidence issue, and that is social anxiety.

Social Anxiety and Lack of Confidence In Specific Situations

Social anxiety is an actual disorder where a person has a phobia in which a person feels like they are being watched and judged by everybody. There may be select situations where this is actually happening, but in most circumstances, it is an unfound fear. This is an extreme situation where a person has a lack of confidence in everything they do, and therefore, feel like they are the center of attention.

Going for a job interview, taking a test, going on a date, or speaking in public are normal things that create anxiety in almost everybody. It is amplified greatly in someone who has a social anxiety disorder. Furthermore, these individuals actually become nervous during normal, everyday activities like shopping for food, parking their car, or using a public restroom. Their anxiety is so intense that they feel judged in every moment of their lives. This fear can become so strong that it interferes with people going to work, attending school, talking to their friends, or doing any other menial task during the day.

It is estimated that about seven percent of the American population suffers from social anxiety. While this number is not massive, it shows that the problem is not uncommon.

Researchers believe there is a genetic component where areas of the brain that deal with fear and anxiety are involved. However, there is no explanation as to why some family members are affected while others are not. For example, out of two siblings, one may be shy and quiet, while the other one is loud and bombastic.

Another cause of social anxiety may be underdeveloped social skills. Some individuals will feel discouraged after talking to people, even if the conversation did not go poorly, which will cause them to avoid interactions in the future. The lack of interaction will just lead to further underdeveloped social skills, and the social anxiety trend will continue.

Many people with this disorder do not have anxiety in specific social settings, but instead in areas where performance is involved. This is often referred to as performance anxiety and is related to performing in front of a crowd in any type of capacity, whether it is a speech, dance recital, or sporting event. Speaking in public is one of the worst fears that people have, and in some surveys, it is number one. Jerry Seinfeld used to make the joke that during a funeral, most people would rather be inside the casket than the ones giving the eulogy.

Even if a person is confident in the subject matter, having to discuss it in a large crowd, with hundreds, or even thousands, of eyes, looking at them, will create a high level of anxiety. This situation would be unsettling for many people. There are many reasons why someone would have a fear of speaking in public, and it goes beyond just being nervous.

Fear and anxiety will create a physiological response within us. During this process, our autonomic nervous system, which works as a protective mechanism by keeping us alert, will make us hyper-arousable. Generally, this is done to put the body in a state of battle. As a result, we will have an emotional experience to fear, which will interfere with our ability to perform well in front of an audience.

Another factor to consider is the person's beliefs about the speaking engagement. Many people will feel that if they screw up something in front of a crowd, it will hurt their credibility, and therefore, their careers. They also feel that their performance will never be forgotten, and their whole public image will be destroyed in an instant. The fact that everyone has a camera on their phones lends some more credibility to this fear. These feelings cause people to overthink and become extremely anxious beyond their control.

Anxiety during a public speech is greater in those who don't do it often. The more a person speaks in front of a crowd, the less nervous they become over time. Unfortunately, most people do not speak in front of audiences constantly, unless they do it for a living. If someone only speaks a few times a year or less, then they will usually have anxiety every time. Also, a person's status in relation to the audience members can play a role in their confidence levels. For example, if a person is speaking in front of high-level executives about a topic they already know, then this can create an immense amount of fear. They worry about having their speech dissected. What a person must realize here is that it is not so much the content of the speech, but how it is presented.

The most obvious reason for the fear of public speaking is the actual skill involved. Speaking in front of an audience involves getting the people engaged. This is done by proper timing, eye contact, stage presences, charisma, and a little bit of humor. The bottom line is, you must be able to connect with the audience somehow, or they will not care whatsoever what you have to say, no matter who you are. Your status may capture their attention for a while, but if you can't keep their attention, your speech will be forgotten before it even starts. Many people know this and are worried that they won't be able to hold their audience's attention.

The more anxious you are, the less likely you are to perform well. It is to your advantage to be as relaxed as possible and overcome your social anxiety, which is much easier said than done.

Aside from public speaking, another social situation that can cause anxiety is being in a large crowd. Many people with social anxiety are okay when they are just around their friends. However, once the circle starts increasing, their anxiety grows tremendously. This type of fear is known as enochlophobia, and it is related to the perceived dangers posed by large gatherings of people you may see in everyday life. The fear includes getting lost, stuck, or harmed in some manner by the crowd.

Most of you are probably thinking of concerts or other places where organized gatherings occur. The simple solution here would be to avoid these types of events. However, this fear also encompasses busy metropolitan areas, public transits like the bus or subway, or even workspaces with a lot of employees. Any type of space where a large number of people are, a person with this type of phobia will become fearful and anxious.

In the next chapter, we will describe various ways to build up your self-confidence, so you can be prepared to handle any situation, even if you are not familiar with it.

Chapter 3: Learning to Become Comfortable

When you lack self-confidence, it means you are unsure of yourself in a particular setting. You have a certain level of discomfort, which precludes you from going all-in when performing a certain task. Unfortunately, if your confidence levels are not high enough, then you will not perform at your highest level. This does not mean you aren't nervous or slightly anxious. It literally means that you do not believe in yourself in a specific situation.

A person will never feel fully confident in every aspect of life. There will be plenty of times when we are faced with something new, and it will completely throw us off our game. The goal of this chapter will be to build self-esteem in some of the most important areas of our lives and also develop the critical thinking skills we need to overcome almost any situation, no matter how unfamiliar it may be.

Building Your Self-Confidence

Nobody is born with an unlimited amount of self-confidence. Also, people are not born with zero confidence. It is something that either gets built-up or deteriorated over time. Unfortunately, many people have had their confidence shattered so many times that they never have confidence in themselves in any situation, no matter how familiar they are with it. The practices in this section will focus on building self-confidence in the general sense, so you are ready to attack life, no matter what gets thrown your way.

Groom Yourself Regularly

This may sound obvious, but many people do not realize how good they will feel when they take the time to shower, do their hair, clean their nails, and dress nicely. The old saying, "When you look good, you feel good," Holds a lot of truth. Even if you have nothing important planned for the day, take the time to groom yourself. You will automatically feel more confident in any situation you come across. You don't have to go to the salon every day or wear thousand-dollar suits. The goal is to look good when you observe yourself in the mirror. This could mean wearing your favorite shirt and jeans combination.

Photoshop Your Self-Image

We take a lot of stock in our self-image. No matter how much we try to say that looks don't matter, we like to look at ourselves in the mirror and see a positive self-image. You can alter your self-image by mentally photoshopping yourself in a way that is positive to you. You can then work on obtaining this image in real-life. For example, if you see yourself 20 pounds lighter, then keep this image in your mind and work towards it.

Destroy Negative Thoughts

No matter how unfamiliar you are with a situation, you are more likely to handle it well if you get rid of your negative thoughts. These simply take up space in your mind and have no value in your productivity. Be aware of our self-talk and how you think about yourself. This may sound ridiculous, but when you find a negative thought entering your mind, picture it as an object or creature that you want to destroy. For example, when you begin having negative thoughts, picture them as bugs. Now, squash those bugs mentally, and you will effectively destroy your negative thoughts. This is a great mental trick to play on yourself. After getting rid of the negative thought, replace it with a positive one.

Get to Know Yourself

When going into battle, it is best to know your enemy very well, no matter who they are. When you are dealing with low self-confidence, your enemy becomes yourself. This is why it is important to get to know yourself as well as you can. Listen intently to your thoughts, write about yourself in a journal, determine what thoughts about yourself dominate your mind, and analyze why you have negative thoughts.

Next, write down all of the positive aspects that you have, no matter how minuscule they may seem. Start thinking about the limitations you have and determine if they are real and verified, or just something you came up with in your head. Dig as deep you can get into your psyche, and you will find out more about yourself than you had ever known. The more you know about yourself, the greater self-confidence you will have.

Be Kind and Generous

Be kind and generous to others, whether it is time, money, or other resources, will be great for improving your self-image. When you are genuinely able to help someone when they need you, then it makes you feel good about who you are. It gives you a sense of purpose.

Be Prepared

Be as prepared for life as you can. Think about this for a moment: if you are taking an exam, and have not studied, then you won't be prepared, and your confidence level will be very low. On the other hand, if you did study intensely, then you will be much more prepared and have a greater amount of confidence. Imagine life as one big exam. The more prepared you are every day, the more confident you will feel in any situation. The following are some general ways you can be more prepared.

- Have plenty of food in the refrigerator and cabinets.
- Have a substantial emergency fund.
- Have the basics as far as emergency supplies at all times.
- If you have something specific planned for that day, like a presentation or meeting, be as prepared as possible for it.
- Always be on alert for dangerous situations.

Know Your Principles and Live By Them

What are the main principles upon which your life is built? If you are not sure, then it's time to sit down and really think about it. Otherwise, your life will be completely directionless. When you know your principles and live by them, then you are truly living your passion, and this is great for your self-confidence. People who are simply coasting through life with no real values will have no goals in life either. They are simply existing and not fully living. When you refuse to live your life based on your values, then you lack confidence in yourself.

Speak Slowly

Speaking slowly will make a huge difference in how people perceive you. It shows a sense of knowledge and confidence in what is being said. Someone who speaks with a rapid-fire approach generally does so because they are not confident in what they are saying. They just want to get the word out there and hope nobody calls them out. Even if you don't feel totally confident on a subject, try speaking slowly anyway, and see how much your self-confidence actually builds. This can be a great mind trick. When you speak slow, you have more time to formulate good thoughts. Of course, I am not telling you to take it to the extreme here, just don't spit words out like a machine gun.

Stand Up Straight

This is another simple trick to help you feel better about yourself. When you slouch, not only does it showcase a lack of confidence, you actually have less self-confidence. This goes along the lines of looking good and feeling good. And trust me, when you stand up straighter, you will look much better.

Increase Your Competence Levels

Simply put, if you are more competent in something, you feel more confident. You gain competence through practice and training. In any situation in life, get as much training as you can to feel as fully self-confident as you can. Let's use the example of a house fire. I hope that your house never burns down, but if it does, I want you to feel confident that you and your family can escape safely. Map out an escape plan and practice it as often as you can. Many companies do quarterly evacuation drills. Employ this same practice in your house. If an emergency like this ever occurs, you will have more competence, and therefore, confidence in being able to handle it. Think of as many possible circumstances as you can in life, and determine ways to practice and train in them.

Set Small Goals and Achieve Them

When you are able to achieve a goal in life, it is a huge boost to your confidence. Set small goals regularly and then work hard to accomplish them. Remember, they should be small and reasonable. You can even cut down larger goals into smaller achievable steps. For example, if your goal is to buy a car, you can create a goal to save a certain amount of money by the end of the month, and then every month after that.

Change Small Habits About Yourself

Trying to change a large habit all at once can be very difficult, and the chances of failure are high. This will be a huge shot to your confidence. Instead, focus on smaller habits that will lead to big change. For example, if your goal is to wake up early and workout before starting your day, then don't try to wake up two hours earlier on the first day. Start by waking up 10-20 minutes early until it becomes a habit, and then increase the time from there as you feel comfortable.

Focus Your Attention on Solutions

So often, we are completely focused on the problems and pay no attention to the solutions. For example, you may always complain about being tired, but do nothing to change it, because the solutions never enter your mind. Make it a habit to focus on solutions whenever a problem enters your mind. You will get more accomplished and gain a lot of self-confidence. For example, if you are tired every day, then what is making you that way. Are you not sleeping enough? If not, then why is that? Are you eating too much sugar before going to bed? Do you have a poor diet during the day? Are you drinking enough water? See how man questions you can get answered if you just shift your focus from the problems to the solutions. Try it out with any small problems that you may have and notice the results.

Become Active

You may have noticed that when you start taking action, work starts getting done. So often, people sit around and worry about how they will get something done, rather than doing the work to get it done. Excessive worry leads to a lack of confidence. The more you worry, the lower your self-confidence will become. If you take action, you will obtain results. Results lead to increased confidence. Next time you find yourself worrying about something, start developing a plan and execute it. Hours of taking actions will give you better results than hours of sitting around and worrying.

Gain More Knowledge

Empowering yourself with knowledge is one of the greatest ways to build self-confidence. You will never know everything, but the more you know, the better you will feel about yourself. This goes along the same vein as building competence. You become more knowledgeable on a subject by studying and practicing it. This does not have to be something you will use. It can just be for your own self-fulfillment. According to psychology, one of the biggest reasons for low self-confidence is either misinformation or a lack of information. As you become more empowered with knowledge, you will gain more information too.

Just like with the steps to gain self-esteem, these previous steps must be employed regularly. Our self-confidence will be challenged all the time, so it is in our best interest to build it up regularly through practice and discipline. Think of your confidence as a muscle that you must work out every single day. Do this, and you will be amazed at how much self-confidence you have throughout your life.

Overcoming Procrastination

People love to procrastinate. And why wouldn't they? Why do something now if you can do it tomorrow? I'll tell you why. What keeps you from making the same excuse tomorrow? Also, how do you know what tomorrow will bring? Perhaps something will happen that prevents you from doing the task then, too. A better question to ask yourself is: Why wait until tomorrow if you can get it done now.

Procrastination is a huge problem in our society, and it leads to a lot of anxiety. This anxiety, in turn, leads to a lack of self-confidence. Procrastination is basically a form of being unprepared. Let's say you have a project due on Friday, and it is now Monday. If you begin working on it now, and do a little bit each day, you will have more confidence in completing the project and doing it well, than you would if you started on Thursday. Imagine how much more thorough you can be by starting projects a little bit earlier. The following are a few easy action steps you can take to help overcome procrastination.

- Do not take on more than you can handle. Keep the number of decisions you have to make to a minimum. The more you have to decide on, the more likely you are to procrastinate.

- Begin focusing on the benefits of completing something, rather than the task. For example, if you are working on a project for work, imagine how good it will feel when it's done. Also, think about the rewards that might come if you perform the task well, like a promotion or raise. This focus on the benefits will give you more motivation to get started.

- Prepare yourself for a task by becoming educated on it. Be aware of your limitations before even picking up a new project and do what you can to obtain the necessary knowledge before moving forward. Once again, knowledge will lead to confidence, and confidence makes you active in a pursuit.

- Turn distractions into rewards. If you cannot get your work done because you are always binge-watching shows, then force yourself to turn them into rewards after a hard day's work. For example, set a timer for three hours and use that time to focus on your projects. After the three hours, pat yourself on the back and watch an episode of the show you like. Remember that you have to stay disciplined.

- Set up a daily schedule system for yourself. For example, the first two hours in the morning are designated for the most important tasks, then a break, followed by two hours of the less important tasks, then another break, and finally, dedicating the last part of the day towards the least important tasks. Once you set up a schedule, stick to it to the best of your ability.

- Avoid getting stuck on a project. Give yourself a certain amount of time on a specific task, and if you cannot make progress, move onto something else and revisit it later. There is no sense in wasting time being nonproductive on something.

Follow these steps religiously and watch procrastination be an afterthought in your life.

Build Confidence At Work

Our jobs are a major part of our lives, and it is important to have self-confidence in this environment. We went over building self-confidence in the general sense earlier in this chapter, and now we will focus on more specific areas in our lives. Many of the action steps and techniques are still the same, while some will be more geared towards work.

- Cut out the negative self-talk. Do not beat yourself up at work. It will do nothing for you. Speaking kindly and encouragingly to yourself and you will learn from whatever mistakes you made more easily.

- Boost your knowledge any way you can, and it is a surefire way to achieve confidence. Stay up on the latest research, services, and products within your company and industry as a whole. Imagine being able to bring an idea to your workplace simply because you read up on it. This will make you feel very good about yourself. Always try to stay ahead of the curve.

- Use opportunities to teach others who know less about a subject than you do. Being able to teach others effectively will boot your own knowledge and confidence.

- Practice what you know incessantly, and always look for ways to improve. Identify and correct mistakes along the way.

- Do not speak poorly about others. This already shows a lack of confidence in yourself. When you compliment and speak highly of other people, you acknowledge their strengths and make them feel good about themselves. In turn, you feel good about yourself, too. This also helps to build a nontoxic work environment.

- Pick up new skills to enhance proficiency at your job.

- Ask questions when you do not know something. You may think that you will feel stupid if you ask a question. However, asking and then doing it right, is a bigger boost to confidence than not asking and screwing things up.

- Eliminate negative language, even if it's not geared at anybody. Negative language can affect our psyche on the deepest levels, effectively lowering our confidence levels without us even realizing it.

- Focus on all of the success you have had at work, rather than the failures.

Chapter 4: Getting Rid of Social Anxiety

Social anxiety encompasses many areas of our lives, such as personal relationships, engaging in activities, hanging out in large groups, or giving public speeches. In order to engage in any of these areas, we must overcome our social anxiety, which is essentially having a lack of confidence in social settings. Depending on the individual, social anxiety will either impact them no matter what setting they're, while for others, it will be more selective. For example, a person may be very talkative and confident among his friends but will be terrified when speaking or performing on stage.

This can be the other way around, too. Legendary late-night host, Johnny Carson, was magnanimous on stage but known to be quiet, reserved, and even shy in small groups. We will go over some basic techniques to improve your social anxiety. These will be effective in just about any setting you are in. These techniques are involved with cognitive behavioral therapy, which is a psychologically-based approach to dealing with anxiety, that is drugfree.

- Think about what you're avoiding. As always, the first step in solving a problem is by identifying what it is. What specific social settings are you avoiding. For instance, some people have stated things like using a public restroom, ordering food at a restaurant, becoming scared in a large group, or speaking up at a meeting. Determine what settings cause your social anxiety. Write these down somewhere so you can keep track.

- Now, take your list that you made and develop some type of rating system. This is used to determine the level of anxiety you might experience in each situation to determine what makes it worse. If you feel the most anxious while giving a public speech, then you can rate that as a 10, and then move down from there. So if being around friends gives you none or very little anxiety, that can be a 0 or 1 rating. These ratings are based mainly on predictions. Basically, we are predicting how we would react in certain social settings.

- The next step is to test your predictions. Go out and put yourself in specific situations that may or may not give you the level of anxiety you predicted. For instance, you may have thought you would be at a level of 9 when meeting someone new at a party, but once you did, it was actually around a 4 rating. You may surprise yourself at how well you can actually cope with your anxiety.

- Identify safety behaviors that you use and work to eliminate them. These are superstitious behaviors that people engage in to make them feel safer. I am not talking about carrying a rabbit's foot. Safety behaviors are things like pre-medicating before a social event, avoiding eye contact, rehearsing what you're going to say, or walking with stiff shoulders. The main problem with these types of behaviors is that you will believe they are the only way to get through an anxiety-casing situation. The more you give up these behaviors, the better your experience will be. Imagine how much better a conversation will be when it's natural, rather than scripted.

- Challenge your anxious thoughts. Instead of thinking about how bad things will go, start thinking about how they will go well. If you are worried about looking foolish, ask yourself why that is, and when have you actually looked foolish in the past? Is it real or made up in your head.

- Practice doing what makes you anxious. The classic example here is giving a speech in front of a mirror or recording yourself while you speak alone in your living room. Remind yourself that people don't usually know what your internal feelings are unless you make it obvious to them. This means that no one may have noticed your anxiety in the past. Eventually, test out what you've practiced in the real world. In the case of a speech, after practicing alone for a while, you can perform it in front of some friends.

- Practice self-reward, rather than post-mortem. Post-mortem means that a person analyzes and criticizes every little thing that they've done during a social encounter. If they were standing awkwardly, they become focused on that. Instead, reward yourself for facing the anxiety-causing situation.

Remember to always rinse and repeat with all of these techniques. They must be done regularly until you develop a pattern. You will never be fully confident in every situation. The world will throw things at you that will make you take a few steps back and throw you off your game. That is okay. The key to these exercises is to build up a certain level of self-confidence so that you will be ready to engage and deal with whatever life throws at you. You will develop true strength and knowledge to overcome, no matter how unfamiliar a situation is.

PART IV

In this chapter, we are going to study the details of the reset diet and what recipes you can make.

Chapter 1: How to Reset Your Body?

Created by a celebrity trainer, Harley Pasternak, the body reset diet is a famous fifteen-day eating pattern that aims to jump-start weight loss. According to Pasternak, if you experience rapid loss in weight early in a diet, you will feel more motivated to stick to that diet plan. This theory is even supported by a few scientific studies (Alice A Gibson, 2017).

The body reset diet claims to help in weight loss with light exercise and low-calorie diet plans for fifteen days. The diet is divided into 3 phases of five days each. Each phase had a particular pattern of diet and exercise routine. You need to consume food five times every day, starting from the first phase, which mostly consists of smoothies and progressing to more solid foods in the second and third phases.

The three phases of the body reset diet are:

- **Phase One** – During this stage, you are required to consume only two snacks every day and drink smoothies for breakfast, lunch, and dinner.

In the case of exercise, you have to walk at least ten thousand steps per day.

- **Phase Two** – During this phase, you can eat two snacks each day, consume solid food only once, and have to replace any two meals of the day with smoothies. In case of exercise, apart from walking ten thousand steps every day, on three of the days, you also have to finish five minutes of resistance training with the help of four separate exercises.

- **Phase Three** – You can consume two snacks every day, but you have to eat two low-calorie meals and replace one of your meals with a smoothie. For exercise, you are required to walk ten thousand steps. Apart from that, you also have to finish five minutes of resistance training with the help of four separate exercises each day.

After you have finished the standard fifteen-day diet requirements, you have to keep following the meal plan you followed in the third phase. However, during this time, you are allowed to have two "free meals" twice a week in which you can consume anything you want. These "free meals" are meant as a reward so that you can avoid feeling deprived. According to Pasternak, depriving yourself of a particular food continuously can result in binge eating (Nawal Alajmi, 2016).

There is no official endpoint of the diet after the first fifteen days for losing and maintaining weight. Pasternak suggests that the habits and routines formed over fifteen days should be maintained for a lifetime.

Chapter 2: Science Behind Metabolism Reset

Several people take on a "cleanse" or "detox" diet every year to lose the extra holiday weight or simply start following healthy habits. However, some fat diet plans are often a bit overwhelming. For example, it requires a tremendous amount of self-discipline to drink only juices. Moreover, even after finishing a grueling detox diet plan, you might just go back to eating foods that are bad for you because of those days of deprivation. New studies issued in the *Medicine & Science in Sports & Exercise* shows that low-calorie diets may result in binge eating, which is not the right method for lasting weight loss.

Another research conducted by the researchers at Loughborough University showed that healthy, college-aged women who followed a calorie-restricted diet consumed an extra three hundred calories at dinner as compared to the control group who consumed three standard meals. They revealed that it was because they had lower levels of peptide YY (represses appetite) and higher levels of ghrelin (makes you hungry). They are most likely to go hog wild when you are feeling ravenous, and it's finally time to eat (Nawal Alajmi K. D.-O., 2016).

Another research published in *Cognitive Neuroscience* studied the brains of chronic dieters. They revealed that there was a weaker connection between the two regions of the brain in people who had a higher percentage of body fat. They showed that they might have an increased risk of getting obese because it's harder for them to set their temptations aside (Pin-Hao Andy Chen, 2016).

A few other studies, however, also revealed that you could increase your self-control through practice. Self-control, similar to any other kind of strength, also requires time to develop. However, you can consider focusing on a diet plan that can help you "reset" instead of putting all your efforts into developing your self-control to get healthy.

A reset is considered as a new start – one that can get your metabolism and your liver in good shape. The liver is the biggest solid organ of your body, and it's mainly responsible for removing toxins that can harm your health and well-being by polluting your system. Toxins keep accumulating in your body all the time, and even though it's the liver's job to handle this, it can sometimes get behind schedule, which can result in inflammation. It causes a lot of strain on your metabolism and results in weight gain, particularly around the abdomen. The best method to alleviate this inflammation is to follow a metabolism rest diet and give your digestive system a vacation (Olivia M. Farr, 2015).

Chapter 3: Recipes for Smoothies and Salads

If you want to lose weight and you have a particular period within which you want to achieve it, then here are some recipes that are going to be helpful.

Green Smoothie

Total Prep & Cooking Time: 2 minutes

Yields: 1 serving

Nutrition Facts: Calories: 144 | Carbs: 28.2g | Protein: 3.4g | Fat: 2.9g | Fiber: 4.8g

Ingredients:

- One cup each of
  - o   Almond milk
  - o   Raw spinach
- One-third of a cup of strawberries
- One orange, peeled

Method:

1. Add the peeled orange, strawberries, almond milk, and raw spinach in a blender and blend everything until you get a smooth paste. You can add extra water if required to achieve the desired thickness.

2. Pour out the smoothie into a glass and serve.

Strawberry Banana Smoothie

Total Prep & Cooking Time: 5 minutes

Yields: 2 servings

Nutrition Facts: Calories: 198| Carbs: 30.8g | Protein: 5.9g | Fat: 7.1g | Fiber: 4.8g

Ingredients:

- Half a cup each of
  - Milk
  - Greek yogurt
- One banana, frozen and quartered
- Two cups of fresh strawberries, halved

Method:

1. Add the milk, Greek yogurt, banana, and strawberries into a high-powered blender and blend until you get a smooth mixture.

2. Pour the smoothie equally into two separate glasses and serve.

Notes:

- *Don't add ice to the smoothie as it can make it watery very quickly. Using frozen bananas will keep your smoothie cold.*

- *As you're using bananas and strawberries, there is no need to add any artificial sweetener.*

Salmon Citrus Salad

Total Prep & Cooking Time: 20 minutes

Yields: 6 servings

Nutrition Facts: Calories: 336 | Carbs: 20g | Protein: 17g | Fat: 21g | Fiber: 5g

Ingredients:

- One pound of Citrus Salmon (slow-roasted)
- Half of an English cucumber, sliced
- One tomato (large), sliced into a quarter of an inch thick pieces
- One grapefruit, peeled and cut into segments
- Two oranges, peeled and cut into segments
- Three beets, roasted and quartered
- One avocado
- Boston lettuce leaves
- Two tablespoons of red wine vinegar
- Half of a red onion
- Flakey salt
- Aleppo pepper flakes

For the Citrus Shallot Vinaigrette,

- Five tablespoons of olive oil (extra-virgin)
- One clove of garlic, smashed

- Salt and pepper
- One and a half tablespoons of rice wine vinegar
- Two tablespoons of orange juice or fresh lemon juice
- One tablespoon of shallot, minced

Method:

For preparing the Citrus Shallot Vinaigrette:

1. Add the ingredients for the vinaigrette in a bowl and whisk them together.

2. Keep the mixture aside.

For assembling the salad,

1. Add the onions and vinegar in a small bowl and pickle them by letting them sit for about fifteen minutes.

2. In the meantime, place the lettuce leaves on the serving plate.

3. Dice the avocado in half and eliminate the pit. Then scoop the flesh and add them onto the plate. Sprinkle a dash of flakey salt and Aleppo pepper on top to season it.

4. Add the quartered beets onto the serving plate along with the grapefruit and orange segments.

5. Salt the cucumber and tomato slices lightly and add them onto the plate.

6. Then, scatter the pickled onions on top and cut the salmon into bits and add it on the plate.

7. Lastly, drizzle the Citrus Shallot Vinaigrette on top of the salad and finish off with a dash of flakey salt.

Chapter 4: Quick and Easy Breakfast and Main Course Recipes

Quinoa Salad

Total Prep & Cooking Time: 40 minutes

Yields: Eight servings

Nutrition Facts: Calories: 205 | Carbs: 25.9g | Protein: 6.1g | Fat: 9.4g | Fiber: 4.6g

Ingredients:

- One tablespoon of red wine vinegar
- One-fourth of a cup each of
    - Lemon juice (about two to three lemons)
    - Olive oil
- One cup each of
    - Quinoa (uncooked), rinsed with the help of a fine-mesh colander
    - Flat-leaf parsley (from a single large bunch), finely chopped
- Three-fourth of a cup of red onion (one small red onion), chopped
- One red bell pepper (medium-sized), chopped
- One cucumber (medium-sized), seeded and chopped
- One and a half cups of chickpeas (cooked), or One can of chickpeas (about fifteen ounces), rinsed and drained

- Two cloves of garlic, minced or pressed

- Two cups of water

- Black pepper, freshly ground

- Half a teaspoon of fine sea salt

Method:

1. Place a medium-sized saucepan over medium-high heat and add the rinsed quinoa into it along with the water. Allow the mixture to boil and then reduce the heat and simmer it. Cook for about fifteen minutes so that the quinoa has absorbed all the water. As time goes on, decrease the heat and maintain a gentle simmer. Take the saucepan away from the heat and cover it with a lid. Allow the cooked quinoa to rest for about five minutes to give it some time to increase in size.

2. Add the onions, bell pepper, cucumber, chickpeas, and parsley in a large serving bowl and mix them together. Keep the mixture aside.

3. Add the garlic, vinegar, lemon juice, olive oil, and salt in another small bowl and whisk the ingredients so that they are appropriately combined. Keep this mixture aside.

4. When the cooked quinoa has almost cooled down, transfer it to the serving bowl. Add the dressing on top and toss to combine everything together.

5. Add an extra pinch of sea salt and the black pepper to season according to your preference. Allow the salad to rest for five to ten minutes before serving it for the best results.

6. You can keep the salad in the refrigerator for up to four days. Make sure to cover it properly.

7. You can serve it at room temperature or chilled.

Notes: Instead of cooking additional quinoa, you can use about three cups of leftover quinoa for making this salad. Moreover, you can also serve this salad with fresh greens and an additional drizzle of lemon juice and olive oil. You can also add a dollop of cashew sour cream or crumbled feta cheese as a topping.

Herb and Goat Cheese Omelet

Total Prep & Cooking Time: 20 minutes

Yields: Two servings

Nutrition Facts: Calories: 233 | Carbs: 3.6g | Protein: 16g | Fat: 17.6g | Fiber: 1g

Ingredients:

- Half a cup each of
  - Red bell peppers (3 x quarter-inch), julienne-cut
  - Zucchini, thinly sliced
- Four large eggs
- Two teaspoons of olive oil, divided
- One-fourth of a cup of goat cheese (one ounce), crumbled
- Half a teaspoon of fresh tarragon, chopped
- One teaspoon each of
  - Fresh parsley, chopped
  - Fresh chives, chopped
- One-eighth of a teaspoon of salt
- One-fourth of a teaspoon of black pepper, freshly ground (divided)
- One tablespoon of water

Method:

1. Break the eggs into a bowl and add one tablespoon of water into it. Whisk them together and add in one-eighth of a teaspoon each of salt and ground black pepper.

2. In another small bowl, mix the goat cheese, tarragon, and parsley and keep it aside.

3. Place a nonstick skillet over medium heat and heat one teaspoon of olive oil in it. Add in the sliced zucchini, bell pepper, and the remaining one-eighth of a teaspoon of black pepper along with a dash of salt. Cook for about four minutes so that the bell pepper and zucchini get soft. Transfer the zucchini-bell pepper mixture onto a plate and cover it with a lid to keep it warm.

4. Add about half a teaspoon of oil into a skillet and add in half of the whisked egg into it. Do not stir the eggs and let the egg set slightly. Loosen the set edges of the omelet carefully with the help of a spatula. Tilt the skillet to move the uncooked part of the egg to the side. Keep following this method for about five seconds so that there is no more runny egg in the skillet. Add half of the crumbled goat cheese mixture evenly over the omelet and let it cook for another minute so that it sets.

5. Transfer the omelet onto a plate and fold it into thirds.

6. Repeat the process with the rest of the egg mixture, half a teaspoon of olive oil, and the goat cheese mixture.

7. Add the chopped chives on top of the omelets and serve with the bell pepper and zucchini mixture.

Mediterranean Cod

Total Prep & Cooking Time: 15 minutes

Yields: 4 servings

Nutrition Facts: Calories: 320 | Carbs: 31g | Protein: 35g | Fat: 8g | Fiber: 8g

Ingredients:

- One pound of spinach
- Four fillets of cod (almost one and a half pounds)
- Two zucchinis (medium-sized), chopped
- One cup of marinara sauce
- One-fourth of a teaspoon of red pepper, crushed
- Two cloves of garlic, chopped
- One tablespoon of olive oil
- Salt and pepper, according to taste
- Whole wheat roll, for serving

Method:

1. Place a ten-inch skillet on medium heat and add the marinara sauce and zucchini into it. Combine them together and let it simmer on medium heat.

2.   Add the fillets of cod into the simmering sauce. Add one-fourth of a teaspoon each of salt and pepper too. Cover the skillet with a lid and let it cook for about seven minutes so that the cod gets just opaque throughout.

3.   In the meantime, place a five-quart saucepot on medium heat and heat the olive oil in it. Add in the crushed red pepper and minced garlic. Stir and cook for about a minute.

4.   Then, add in the spinach along with one-eighth of a teaspoon of salt. Cover the saucepot with a lid and let it cook for about five minutes, occasionally stirring so that the spinach gets wilted.

5.   Add the spinach on the plates and top with the sauce and cod mixture and serve with the whole wheat roll.

Grilled Chicken and Veggies

Total Prep & Cooking Time: 35 minutes

Yields: 4 servings

Nutrition Facts: Calories: 305 | Carbs: 11g | Protein: 26g | Fat: 17g | Fiber: 3g

Ingredients:

For the marinade,

- Four cloves of garlic, crushed
- One-fourth of a cup each of
  o Fresh lemon juice
  o Olive oil
- One teaspoon each of
  o Salt
  o Smoked paprika
  o Dried oregano
- Black pepper, according to taste
- Half a teaspoon of red chili flakes

For the grilling,

- Two to three zucchinis or courgette (large), cut into thin slices
- Twelve to sixteen spears of asparagus, woody sides trimmed
- Broccoli

- Two bell peppers, seeds eliminated and cut into thin slices
- Four pieces of chicken breasts (large), skinless and de-boned

Method:

1. Preheat your griddle or grill pan.

2. Sprinkle some salt on top of the chicken breasts to season them. Keep them aside to rest while you prepare the marinade.

3. For the marinade, mix all the ingredients properly.

4. Add about half of the marinade over the vegetables and the other half over the seasoned chicken breasts. Allow the marinade to rest for a couple of minutes.

5. Place the chicken pieces on the preheated grill. Grill for about five to seven minutes on each side until they are cooked according to your preference. The time on the grill depends on the thickness of the chicken breasts.

6. Remove them from the grill and cover them using a foil. Set it aside to rest and prepare to grill the vegetables in the meantime.

7. Grill the vegetables for a few minutes until they begin to char and are crispy yet tender.

8. Remove them from the grill and transfer them onto a serving plate. Serve the veggies along with the grilled chicken and add the lemon wedges on the side for squeezing.

Notes: You can add as much or as little vegetables as you like. The vegetable amounts are given only as a guide. Moreover, feel free to replace some of them with the vegetables you like to eat.

Stuffed Peppers

Total Prep & Cooking Time: 50 minutes

Yields: 4 servings

Nutrition Facts: Calories: 438 | Carbs: 32g | Protein: 32g | Fat: 20g | Fiber: 5g

Ingredients:

For the stuffed peppers,

- One pound of ground chicken or turkey
- Four bell peppers (large) of any color
- One and a quarter of a cups of cheese, shredded
- One and a half cups of brown rice, cooked (you can use cauliflower rice or quinoa)
- One can (about fourteen ounces) of fire-roasted diced tomatoes along with its juices
- Two teaspoons of olive oil (extra-virgin)
- One teaspoon each of
  o Garlic powder
  o Ground cumin
- One tablespoon of ground chili powder
- One-fourth of a teaspoon of black pepper
- Half a teaspoon of kosher salt

For serving,

- Sour cream or Greek yogurt

- Salsa

- Freshly chopped cilantro

- Avocado, sliced

- Freshly squeezed lemon juice

Method:

1. Preheat your oven to 375 degrees Fahrenheit.

2. Take a nine by thirteen-inch baking dish and coat it lightly with a nonstick cooking spray.

3. Take the bell peppers and slice them from top to bottom into halves. Remove the membranes and the seeds. Keep the bell peppers in the baking dish with the cut-side facing upwards.

4. Place a large, nonstick skillet on medium-high heat and heat the olive oil in it. Add in the chicken, pepper, salt, garlic powder, ground cumin, and chili powder and cook for about four minutes so that the chicken is cooked through and gets brown. Break apart the chicken while it's cooking. Drain off any excess liquid and then add in the can of diced tomatoes along with the juices. Allow it to simmer for a minute.

5. Take the pan away from the heat. Add in the cooked rice along with three-fourth of a cup of the shredded cheese and stir everything together.

6. Add this filling inside the peppers and add the remaining shredded cheese as a topping.

7. Add a little amount of water into the pan containing the peppers so that it barely covers the bottom of the pan.

8. Keep it uncovered and bake it in the oven for twenty-five to thirty-five minutes so that the cheese gets melted and the peppers get soft.

9. Add any of your favorite fixings as a topping and serve hot.

Notes:

- *For preparing the stuffed peppers ahead of time, make sure to allow the rice and chicken mixture to cool down completely before filling the peppers. You can prepare the stuffed peppers before time, and then you have to cover it with a lid and keep it in the refrigerator for a maximum of twenty-four hours before baking the peppers.*

- *If you're planning to reheat the stuffed peppers, gently reheat them in your oven or microwave. If you're using a microwave for this purpose, make sure to cut the peppers into pieces to warm them evenly.*

- *You can store any leftovers in the freezer for up to three months. Alternatively, you can keep them in the refrigerator for up to four days. Allow it to thaw in the fridge overnight.*

Brussels Sprouts With Honey Mustard Chicken

Total Prep & Cooking Time: Fifty minutes

Yields: Four servings

Nutrition Facts: Calories: 360 | Carbs: 14.5g | Protein: 30.8g | Fat: 20g | Fiber: 3.7g

Ingredients:

- One and a half pounds of Brussels sprouts, divided into two halves
- Two pounds of chicken thighs, skin-on and bone-in (about four medium-sized thighs)
- Three cloves of garlic, minced
- One-fourth of a large onion, cut into slices
- One tablespoon each of
    o Honey
    o Whole-grain mustard
    o Dijon mustard
- Two tablespoons of freshly squeezed lemon juice (one lemon)
- One-fourth of a cup plus two tablespoons of olive oil (extra-virgin)
- Freshly ground black pepper
- Kosher salt
- Non-stick cooking spray

Method:

1. Preheat your oven to 425 degrees Fahrenheit.

2. Take a large baking sheet and grease it with nonstick cooking spray. Keep it aside.

3. Add the minced garlic, honey, whole-grain mustard, Dijon mustard, one tablespoon of the lemon juice, one-fourth cup of the olive oil in a medium-sized bowl and mix them together. Add the Kosher salt and black pepper to season according to your preference.

4. Dip the chicken thighs into the sauce with the help of tongs and coat both sides. Transfer the things on the baking sheet. You can get rid of any extra sauce.

5. Mix the red onion and Brussels sprouts in a medium-sized bowl and drizzle one tablespoon of lemon juice along with the remaining two tablespoons of olive oil onto it. Toss everything together until the vegetables are adequately coated.

6. Place the red onion-Brussels sprouts mixture on the baking sheet around the chicken pieces. Ensure that the chicken and vegetables are not overlapping.

7. Sprinkle a little amount of salt and pepper on the top and keep it in the oven to roast for about thirty to thirty-five minutes so that the Brussels sprouts get crispy and the chicken has an internal temperature of 165 degrees Fahrenheit and has turned golden brown.

8. Serve hot.

Quinoa Stuffed Chicken

Total Prep & Cooking Time: 50 minutes

Yields: Four servings

Nutrition Facts: Calories: 355 | Carbs: 28g | Protein: 30g | Fat: 13g | Fiber: 4g

Ingredients:

- One and a half cups of chicken broth
- Three-fourths of a cup of quinoa (any color of your choice)
- Four chicken breasts (boneless and skinless)
- One lime, zested and one tablespoon of lime juice
- One-fourth of a cup of cilantro, chipped
- One-third of a cup of unsweetened coconut, shaved or coconut chips
- One Serrano pepper, seeded and diced
- Two cloves of garlic, minced
- Half a cup of red onion, diced
- Three-fourth of a cup of bell pepper, diced
- One tablespoon of coconut oil
- One teaspoon each of
  - Salt
  - Chili powder
  - Ground cumin

Method:

1. Preheat your oven to 375 degrees Fahrenheit.

2. Take a rimmed baking sheet and line it with parchment paper.

3. Place a medium-sized saucepan over medium-high heat and add the coconut oil in it. After it has melted, add in the Serrano peppers, garlic, red onion, and bell pepper and sauté for about one to two minutes so that they soften just a bit. Make sure that the vegetables are still bright in color. Then transfer the cooked vegetables into a bowl.

4. Add the quinoa in the empty sauce pot and increase the heat to high. Pour the chicken broth in it along with half a teaspoon of salt. Close the lid of the pot and bring it to a boil, allowing the quinoa to cook for about fifteen minutes so that the surface of the quinoa develops vent holes, and the broth has absorbed completely. Take the pot away from the heat and allow it to steam for an additional five minutes.

5. In the meantime, cut a slit along the long side in each chicken breast. It will be easier with the help of a boning knife. You are making a deep pocket in each breast, having a half-inch border around the remaining three attached sides. Keep the knife parallel to the cutting board and cut through the middle of the breast and leaving the opposite side attached. Try to cut it evenly as it's challenging to cook thick uncut portions properly in the oven. After that, add salt, cumin, and chili powder on all sides of the chicken.

6. When the quinoa has turned fluffy, add in the lime juice, lime zest, shaved coconut, and sautéed vegetables and stir them in. Taste the mixture and adjust the salt as per your preference.

7. Add the confetti quinoa mixture inside the cavity of the chicken breast. Place the stuffed breasts on the baking sheet with the quinoa facing upwards. They'll look like open envelopes.

8. Bake them in the oven for about twenty minutes.

9. Serve warm.

Kale and Sweet Potato Frittata

Total Prep & Cooking Time: 30 minutes

Yields: 4 servings

Nutrition Facts: Calories: 144 | Carbs: 10g | Protein: 7g | Fat: 9g | Fiber: 2g

Ingredients:

- Three ounces of goat cheese
- Two cloves of garlic
- Half of a red onion (small)
- Two cups each of
  - Sweet potatoes
  - Firmly packed kale, chopped
- Two tablespoons of olive oil
- One cup of half-and-half
- Six large eggs
- Half a teaspoon of pepper, freshly ground
- One teaspoon of Kosher salt

Method:

1. Preheat your oven to 350 degrees Fahrenheit.

2. Add the eggs, half-and-half, salt, and black pepper in a bowl and whisk everything together.

3. Place a ten-inch ovenproof nonstick skillet over medium heat and add one tablespoon of oil in it. Sauté the sweet potatoes in the skillet for about eight to ten minutes so that they turn soft and golden brown. Transfer them onto a plate and keep warm.

4. Next, add in the remaining one tablespoon of oil and sauté the kale along with the red onions and garlic in it for about three to four minutes so that the kale gets soft and wilted. Then, add in the whisked egg mixture evenly over the vegetables and cook for an additional three minutes.

5. Add some goat cheese on the top and bake it in the oven for ten to fourteen minutes so that it sets.

Walnut, Ginger, and Pineapple Oatmeal

Total Prep & Cooking Time: 30 minutes

Yields: 4 servings

Nutrition Facts: Calories: 323 | Carbs: 61g | Protein: 6g | Fat: 8g | Fiber: 5g

Ingredients:

- Two large eggs
- Two cups each of
  - Fresh pineapple, coarsely chopped
  - Old-fashioned rolled oats
  - Whole milk
- One cup of walnuts, chopped
- Half a cup of maple syrup
- One piece of ginger
- Two teaspoons of vanilla extract
- Half a teaspoon of salt

Method:

1. Preheat your oven to 400 degrees Fahrenheit.

2.   Add the ginger, walnuts, pineapple, oats, and salt in a large bowl and mix them together. Add the mixture evenly among four ten-ounce ramekins and keep them aside.

3.   Whisk the eggs along with the milk, maple syrup, and vanilla extract in a medium-sized bowl. Pour one-quarter of this mixture into each ramekin containing the oat-pineapple mixture.

4.   Keep the ramekins on the baking sheet and bake them in the oven for about twenty-five minutes until the oats turn light golden brown on the top and have set properly.

5.   Serve with some additional maple syrup on the side.

Caprese Salad

Total Prep & Cooking Time: 15 minutes

Yields: 4 servings

Nutrition Facts: Calories: 216 | Carbs: 4g | Protein: 13g | Fat: 16g | Fiber: 1g

Ingredients:

For the salad,

- Nine basil leaves (medium-sized)
- Eight ounces of fresh whole-milk mozzarella cheese
- Two tomatoes (medium-sized)
- One-fourth of a teaspoon of black pepper, freshly ground
- Half a teaspoon of Kosher salt, or one-fourth of a teaspoon of sea salt

For the dressing,

- One teaspoon of Dijon mustard
- One tablespoon each of
  - Balsamic vinegar
  - Olive oil

Method:

1. Add the olive oil, balsamic vinegar, and Dijon mustard into a small bowl and whisk them together with the help of a small hand whisk so that you get a smooth salad dressing. Keep it aside.

2. Cut the tomatoes into thin slices and try to get ten slices in total.

3. Cut the mozzarella into nine thin slices with the help of a sharp knife.

4. Place the slices of tomatoes and mozzarella on a serving plate, alternating and overlapping one another. Then, add the basil leaves on the top.

5. Season the salad with black pepper and salt and drizzle the prepared dressing on top.

6. Serve immediately.

One-Pot Chicken Soup

Total Prep & Cooking Time: 30 minutes

Yields: 6 servings

Nutrition Facts: Calories: 201 | Carbs: 20g | Protein: 16g | Fat: 7g | Fiber: 16g

Ingredients:

- Three cups of loosely packed chopped kale (or other greens of your choice)
- Two cups of chicken, shredded
- One can of white beans (about fifteen ounces), slightly drained
- Eight cups of broth (vegetable broth or chicken broth)
- Four cloves of garlic, minced
- One cup of yellow or white onion, diced
- One tablespoon of avocado oil (skip if you are using bacon)
- One strip of uncured bacon, chopped (optional)
- Black pepper + sea salt, according to taste

Method:

1. Place a Dutch oven or a large pot over medium heat. When it gets hot, add in the oil or bacon (optional), stirring occasionally, and allow it to get hot for about a minute.

2. Then, add in the diced onion and sauté for four to five minutes, occasionally stirring so that the onions get fragrant and translucent. Add in the minced garlic next and sauté for another two to three minutes. Be careful so as not to burn the ingredients.

3. Then, add the chicken, slightly drained white beans, and broth and bring the mixture to a simmer. Cook for about ten minutes to bring out all the flavors. Taste the mixture and add salt and pepper to season according to your preference. Add in the chopped kale in the last few minutes of cooking. Cover the pot and let it cook until the kale has wilted.

4. Serve hot.

Notes: You can store any leftovers in the freezer for up to a month. Or, you can store them in the refrigerator for a maximum of three to four days. Simply reheat on the stovetop or in the microwave and eat it later.

Chocolate Pomegranate Truffles

Total Prep & Cooking Time: 10 minutes

Yields: Twelve to Fourteen truffles

Nutrition Facts: Calories: 95 | Carbs: 26g | Protein: 1g | Fat: 2g | Fiber: 3g

Ingredients:

- One-third of a cup of pomegranate arils
- Half a teaspoon each of
  - Vanilla extract
  - Ground cinnamon
- Half a cup of ground flax seed
- Two tablespoons of cocoa powder (unsweetened)
- About one tablespoon of water
- One and a half cups of pitted Medjool dates
- One-eighth of a teaspoon of salt

Method:

1. Add the pitted dates in a food processor and blend until it begins to form a ball. Add some water and pulse again. Add in the vanilla, cinnamon, flax seeds, cocoa powder, and salt and blend until everything is combined properly.

2. Turn off the food processor and unplug it. Add in the pomegranate arils and fold them in the mixture so that they are distributed evenly.

3. Make twelve to fourteen balls using the mixture. You can create an outer coating or topping if you want by rolling the balls in finely shredded coconut or cocoa powder.

Notes: *You can store the chocolate pomegranate truffles in the fridge in an air-tight container for a maximum of three days.*

PART V

Chapter 1: Self-Esteem and Valuing Yourself

Imagine waking up in the morning and being full of life. You are energetic as you get out of bed and are ready to attack the day because nothing can stop you. Any type of challenge that comes your way, you are prepared to face it head-on and overcome it. You take pride in your work and relationships because you understand their worth. You also understand the value that you bring to the day, so you carry yourself with strength and dignity.

On the other hand, picture yourself waking up in a crummy mood. You are not looking forward to the day ahead, and no matter what good things may come, they are quickly tossed aside, and your mind wanders towards the negative side. You suffer from anxiety throughout the day, and you avoid any challenging situation you can because you lack faith in yourself.

These two mindsets are entirely different from one another, but they are related to the same thing: Your self-esteem. Self-esteem is the amount of respect that you place on yourself. It is how much you value your skills and ability to handle life and all its circumstances. Those who place a high value on themselves have a high level of self-esteem. Those who set a low value on themselves suffer from low self-esteem.

Your self-esteem is also your self-worth, and you mustn't put a low price tag on your abilities.

Having high self-esteem does not mean you ignore your flaws. It means that you love yourself despite all of them. You recognize your weaknesses, and therefore, are more likely to fix them. In the end, you love yourself because of your own self-beliefs.

As we grow up, we are constantly surrounded by things that affect our psyche. Our ego is the part of our mind that has a direct relationship with the outside world. When we experience an event or interact with a specific individual, it will determine how we feel at that exact moment. If the situation is upsetting, then it can bring out a range of different emotions in us. For those who are dealing with low self-esteem, they will easily be triggered by an outside event. For example, if someone calls us a negative name, it might make us feel sad or angry. This one incident could ruin our whole day in an instant. If we are experiencing negativity over a long period of time, then these thoughts will slowly enter into our subconscious and unconscious mind, where they stay forever, unless we purposefully remove them.

If you have a healthy level of self-esteem, then these situations will roll off your back. Negative people or situations will not change the feelings you have towards yourself because you will be in complete control of your emotions. I am not suggesting that being insulted will not be hurtful for this type of individual, but they will understand how to manage it and not let it affect them negatively. They don't define themselves by other people's opinions.

I can talk all day about the extreme benefits of self-esteem, as there are many. The focus of this book, though, is how to develop and build your self-esteem, even if you have been suffering from low levels of it your whole life. I am working off the assumption that you are in the camp of low self-esteem. Therefore, you already know how it feels, because you are personally living it.

How Low Self-Esteem Is Developed

The first step in dealing with low self-esteem is recognizing that you have it. Now that we have established that, it is important to determine why you have low self-esteem.

The Different Types of Parents

One of the major contributing factors to our self-esteem is our parents and how they raised us. Our mother and father are generally the first people we become close to. How they interact with us will initially determine how we value ourselves. Even if a parent is loving, there are still specific tendencies that can be counterproductive to use raising our self-worth.

While parents often push their children to succeed, some can become overbearing to the point where they use ridicule, harsh criticisms, and even abuse to ensure their children stay on the straight path. While some parents do not have malicious intent when they become disapproving authority figures, others will purposefully look down on their kids and make them feel inferior. Children who grow up under these conditions grow into adults who are never comfortable in their own skin.

On the opposite end of the overbearing caregiver is the uninvolved caregiver who does not care one bit. They ignore their children as if they are not necessary. In fairness, this can often be done unintentionally. For example, the parents work so much and become excessively focused on their jobs. They are obsessed with making a living and ignore the people closest to them, including their children. When children get ignored by the influential adults in their lives, they become confused about their place in the world. They feel forgotten and unimportant, and therefore, they believe their existence to be bothersome to people.

Another parental issue that affects children is the parents or caregivers who are in constant conflict. When these adults fight and throw hurtful language at one another, especially in front of children, they absorb these negative emotions. These children can feel like they contributed to the fighting in some way. Growing into adulthood, these same children will feel like they are the cause of so many different conflicts, simply because they were nearby.

Bullying

Bullying has been an issue for children and adults alike for generations. The powerful always seem to push around the weak. With children, this power is usually in the form of physical dominance. The bigger and stronger child picks on the smaller and weaker one. Of course, the bullying can be mental or psychological, too, if the child can pull it off.

Bullying can also become a significant contributor to low self-esteem. A child who is constantly bullied in any way will develop a poor self-image about themselves. Unfortunately, bullying will never go away. What matters in these situations is the support that children receive from their parents. The way the adults in a child's life handle the aftermath of bullying will play a major role in their mindset development.

Many children do not have a comforting environment to come home to, which is detrimental to their psyche. After experiencing abuse outside the come, they walk through their front door and experience even more of it. This makes a child feel worthless and abandoned. They become lost further into the abyss and think they do not belong anywhere. Having unsupportive parents will magnify the effects of bullying.

Furthermore, some parents were over-supportive. These are the ones who coddled their children and gave them no coping skills to deal with the outside world. As a result, they will be ill-prepared to deal with the cruel world that exists out there, which is not going away anytime soon. When children become adults and enter the real world, they will face some harsh criticisms that will challenge their beliefs about who they are. If they were always buttered up as children, they would not understand how to face rejection, insults, or people being mean to them.

No parent wants their children to feel bad, but they cannot be shielded from disappointment their whole lives. Once they do face this disappointment in the real world, they will fall apart because they have no actual self-worth. All of their value is tied to the compliments that other people give them.

I know I have been singling out parents here, and that's because they are the adults a child spends the most amount of time with. However, other adults, like extended family members, teachers, coaches, or counselors, can also do their part in providing a supportive atmosphere for the children in their lives.

Trauma

Trauma can be physical, emotional, or sexual, and no matter what kind you were a victim of, it will devastate your self-esteem, especially as a child. With trauma, you are being forced into a position against your will, which makes you feel like you've lost power and control of your situation.

Situations like this will make you feel worthless. You will even blame yourself for causing the trauma or abuse. This is a method many people use to gain control back into their lives. They believe that by taking the blame, they will be able to manage the situation the next time it comes around

Children do not have control over who is in their lives. This means they are often stuck in abusive situations and have no way of getting out of it. If they are lucky, someone will recognize it, and they will help them get out.

A child who goes through trauma will grow into an adult who is unsure of themselves in many ways. They will never feel like they are good enough, will always feel like they are to blame for specific situations, and will have a distrust for humanity in general.

I know I have spoken about a lack of trust throughout this book. A significant part of having self-esteem is being able to put your faith into the unknown. When you lack trust, this faith does not exist, and therefore, you will always be paranoid and never fully confident in any situation.

Now, think back on your life and determine the traumatic events you may have gone through. How did these affect your psyche at that moment? How you felt on the inside when these various circumstances occurred will help you understand if they contributed to a lack of self-esteem.

We went over these issues simply to help you recognize the underlying causes of the value you place on yourself. There is nothing we can do about these situations now, but we can learn from them and work on ways to overcome our mental blocks to positive self-esteem.

The Science of Self-Esteem

There has been a lot of research done on the genetic components of low self-esteem. While people can be born with certain levels of chemicals that influence their emotions and brain activity, there is no conclusive evidence that people are born with high or low self-esteem. Even twins who grew up in different environments were found to have different qualities related to their self-worth, even though various other personality traits were similar. As of now, environmental factors seem to play a much more significant role.

Of course, this does not mean that there is no scientific component to all of this. As we go through various life stages, our brain development occurs based on life experiences. The actions we take and the thoughts we create make numerous neural pathways in our brain and nervous system, which determine our future behavior. For example, if we continuously have negative feelings, our mind becomes wired in a certain way to produce these same thoughts in the future. As a result, you habitually think negatively in every situation you come across.

Now that we have established what low self-esteem is, our goal in the next chapter is to help you rewire your brain, so you can start living with high self-esteem.

Chapter 2: How You Can Matter to Yourself

"Confront the dark parts of yourself, and work to banish them with illumination and forgiveness. Your willingness to wrestle with your demons will cause your angels to sing."

-August Summer

Now that we know what self-esteem is, it is hard to deny the role it plays in our lives. Any type of pursuit, whether personal, professional, relationships, or health, will require you to place a high value on yourself; otherwise, you will never progress forward as you should. At this moment, I want you to recognize the past mistakes that brought you to where you are now, but also forgive yourself for them because you can do nothing to change the past. You can learn from it, though, and build a new future where you actually value yourself and the gifts you bring to the world.

In the previous chapter, we discussed the numerous causes of low self-esteem, many of which stem from our childhood. Since our mindset took a long time to develop, it will take extreme effort with several actionable steps to change and overcome this thought-process. We will now discuss some specific steps and practices over the next few chapters you can engage in to improve your mindset and build-up your self-esteem.

We will approach this subject from many different aspects, so they can be combined to improve how you habitually think about yourself. Think of your mind as a structure that is built to think a specific way. Now imagine having to rebuild many different parts of that structure to change your thoughts. This is what we will be doing with all of the action steps we will go over.

How to Build Self-Awareness

Self-awareness means having the ability to understand the way you think, feel, and behave. This is a necessary quality to have if you want to fix your self-esteem. It is the best way to recognize if your actions correlate with low self-esteem. Once you become self-aware, you will know yourself much better. The following are some significant strategies you can employ right away.

Recognize What Bothers You About Other People

What bothers us most about other people are often the same qualities that we possess. For example, if someone is naturally aggressive, we may dislike it; however, it is a trait that we have, as well. We all have aspects of our personality that are unflattering, and since we don't want to admit them, we will ignore them fully. Ignorance is not bliss in the long-run, and if we do not pay attention to our negative qualities, they will rear their ugly heads at the most inopportune time. The next time a person is bothering you, stop and ask yourself if they are displaying something that is a reflection of you. Do you recognize their personality when you look in the mirror?

Meditate on Your Mind

Mindful meditation is a great way to learn about your thoughts and how they work. One of the main reasons we lack self-awareness is because we are thinking so much that our thoughts completely take over. Proper meditation allows us to separate ourselves from these thoughts and recognize that they do not fully encompass who we are. Through mindful meditation practices, you have the ability to observe your thoughts without becoming attached to them. Therefore, it is easier to see which ones deserve our attention and which ones do not. The following are some simple steps to get you started on this practice.

- Get comfortable by finding a quiet place that is as free from distractions as possible.
- Sit up with your back straight and chest out. It does not matter if you are in a chair or sitting cross-legged on the floor. You may even lie down flat on the floor.
- Take in some deep breaths through your nose and then out slowly through your mouth or nose. You should be able to feel the breaths down into your abdomen. This will help you relax.
- Pay attention to the sounds of your breaths and their rhythmic patterns. When you inhale, imagine breathing in joy and peace. When you breathe out, imagine getting rid of the toxicity in your mind.
- When you notice your thoughts wandering away from your breaths, immediately focus them back to the center. Take in your

immediate surroundings and be in your present state. Do not think of the past or worry about the future.

- Make this practice a habit and do it routinely. Some of the best practitioners of mindful meditation have been doing it for years, and are still learning better ways to improve. These are all great steps to get you started and reorganize your mind.

As a side note, meditation is not only useful for self-awareness. It can help with stress and anxiety, communication, better sleep, improved focus on your goals, and overall mental health. All of this will lead back to higher self-esteem. Start off with five minutes and then build yourself up to 20-30. You will be amazed at how much clarity you will have about yourself.

Draw a Timeline of Your Life

Sit down with a notepad and try to remember as much as you can from the time of birth to where you are now. Pay special attention to significant moments that had a big impact on your life and circumstances, whether positive or negative. This practice will allow you to see certain moments of your life in context, which will give you a better idea of who you are. You will realize a lot about yourself and gain much self-awareness.

Identify Your Emotional Kryptonite

Think about the emotions that you absolutely hate having and try to avoid. For example, some individuals hate feeling sad so much that they drown this emotion with alcohol. The problem is, negative emotions are a gateway into our souls. They are trying to tell us something in a discrete way. If we pay attention to them as they are happening, we will learn a lot about our situation. If you are sad often, pay attention to why so you can finally address it.

Travel and Get Out a Little Bit

We often become stuck in our own little box and forget that there is a big world out there. Micro-travel, which means traveling to new destinations that are local to us, is a great way to get you out of your comfort zone and try out a new routine. Take frequent short trips if you can, and even travel abroad if this is feasible. This will help you gain a lot of awareness for the world around you, as well as teach you a lot about yourself. Travel to new destinations, even nearby, will significantly raise our self-awareness.

Pick Up a New Skill

Just like with travel, learning a new skill will force us to think and act in new ways, thereby forcing us to increase our self-awareness. We all develop certain routines as we grow older, and it causes us to go into a comfort zone. The main problem here is that it creates a strong, narrow-mindedness. Being willing to start something as a beginner will cultivate a level of flexibility in our minds and thoughts. The new skill does not have to be related to your career. It can also be hobbies like playing the piano, sculpting, or dancing.

Clarify Your True Values

How often do you sit down and assess what your true values are? If you are like most people, probably very seldomly. We often get so caught up in daily life that we have very little time for self-reflection, especially on the important things in life. As a result, we end up chasing false goals and not living the type of life we want to. People become so worried about moving up the career ladder and buying the latest fancy car, that they forget what actually makes them happy. In your case, you may have followed a safe career path rather than focus on what your true calling was.

A great technique you can perform is to set aside some time on a weekly or monthly basis and think about your life and circumstances. Ask yourself why you think you are here and what your purpose in life is? Also, imagine what a fulfilling life would look like for you. Spend about 30 minutes every time you do this. A major part of self-awareness is recognizing what really matters to you. This practice will be a great way to come to this understanding.

We tend to get lost in the monotony of life. So, it is important to practice these self-awareness techniques on a regular basis. Taking notice of your thoughts, behaviors, and actions in real-time is a special skill to have. It will go a long way in helping you build your self-esteem.

Chapter 3: Creating a Stronger Self

Going along the path of improved self-esteem, I will now discuss various strategies to strengthen your psyche. High self-esteem requires a strong mindset.

Managing Your Ego

I spoke briefly in chapter one about the ego. Our ego is basically our mind's direct connection to the outside world. What our environment gives, our ego responds. This means that whatever activities are going on around will make you feel a certain way, and this is directly the result based on how our ego responds. For example, if someone outshines us in some way, our ego will respond by making us feel inferior.

People who are not careful will have this aspect of the mind completely control them. As a result, the values they place on themselves are based on what the world thinks of them, rather than what they think of themselves. Every one of us has an ego to a certain degree, but the key is to not let it control us. We must learn to manage it properly so that our self-worth comes from within, rather than from what we can't control. The following are specific steps you can take to begin managing your ego so that it doesn't control you.

Don't Take Things Personally

Taking things too personally or literally can make you overthink and cause your mind to become infected. It's important to be at peace with yourself and realize that people do not always mean what they say. They are often angry or suffering from some other negative emotion. Even if they do mean it, people who treat others poorly have a problem within themselves, and not necessarily other people. In a moment where you are facing harsh words or actions, imagine your spot being replaced by someone else and watching the same people act in the same manner because, in most cases, they would. A big part of self-esteem is not caring what others think. This is a major step in that direction.

Accepts All of Your Mistakes

Accepting your mistakes, no matter how big or small is a positive way to work on your ego problems. Everyone makes mistakes, so there is no use in hiding them. Once you admit them, apologize, and move on, they no longer have control over you as you've released them from your psyche. Genuinely apologizing to someone is a great way to put your ego in check and grow as a person.

Stop Being Self-Conscious

Our ego prevents us from looking silly or goofy. We are so afraid of what others are thinking that we never let out guard down. This is a real definition of living in fear. If you have been acting this way for a while, then it's time to stop putting up a shield, and just let your silly self come out. You will actually be happier in the long run because showcasing your true self will attract your real friends. To stop being so self-conscious, try using the following steps.

- Shrug away your negative thoughts. This does not mean you should ignore them. Acknowledge that they are there, but then do not agree with them in any way.

- Don't put other people on pedestals. We have a tendency to do this, especially to those who we admire. Realize that they are regular people and not someone to bow down to.

- Think of a moment where you were self-conscious, and then imagine replacing yourself with someone you cared about in the position. If they felt the same way you did, then what would you tell them. Now, tell that same thing to yourself. We are often bigger critics of ourselves than we are other people.

- Accept yourself, with your faults and all. Remember that nobody is perfect, and if you want to gain a high level of self-esteem, then you must learn to love yourself, including your flaws.

- People are not paying as much attention to you as you may think. Part of our ego tells us that people are watching us and critiquing our every move. Understand that people are in their own world much of the time, and too busy in their personal self-doubts to pay attention to anyone else. Believe it or not, you are not the focus of attention all the time.

- Go do the thing that makes you self-conscious or nervous. Face it head-on, and you will realize it's not as bad as you may think. Do not let your awkwardness keep you on the sidelines. Jump in with both feet and dare to look foolish. If you hate dancing in front of people, join a dance class and do it several times a week. If you suck at basketball, go to the part and shoot hoops in front of people.

Realize That Your Ego Will Never Go Away

Controlling and managing your ego will have to become a routine in your life. It will never fully go away and will rear its ugly head at the most inopportune times if you let your guard down. Always be on high alert of your ego trying to take over, and you will continue to overcome it.

You Are Not the Best

I am not trying to be insulting here, but knowing that you are not going to be the best in every situation means that you understand your limitations. Everyone has limitations, so there is no sense in feeling bad over them. Accept that you are not perfect, but recognize that it does mean you cannot accomplish your goals. You may just need to work harder and focus more on certain areas.

Imagine Your Ego as Another Person

This step may seem ridiculous, but imagine your ego as another person. It is best to picture someone that you may listen, but never actually take advice from, like a whining child. Now, once you imagine your ego in this manner, allow it to speak and say what it needs, acknowledge it with a "thank you," and then move on. When you can actually picture your ego in this way, it will do a lot in stopping you from making significant mistakes.

Stop Bragging

There is no need to brag about your accomplishments. If they are great enough, other people will do the talking for you. The less you talk about yourself, the more humble you become, and humility is a major aspect of self-esteem. You never feel the need to talk yourself up.

Be Grateful for the Little Things

Gratitude is great for improving your attitude. When you start being grateful for the little things, you do not worry so much about the big things. Also, remember that some people cannot have what you have, no matter how hard they try. With the same token, some people will be in a different position than you, that you are unable to reach. That is okay. Just focus on yourself and what you have.

Learn to Compliment Others

People with large egos have a hard time admitting when others have done a great job. They feel it will take the spotlight off of them. Practicing paying even the smallest compliments to other people can help you take the attention off of your ego problems.

On top of these practices, we have gone over, a few other ways to get rid of your ego include:

- Embrace a beginner's attitude. Try something new regularly that forces you to challenge yourself. This will help you realize that you are not perfect at everything.

- Concentrate on the effort you put in, and not the results. You will be forced to see how much you put into an activity, and determine if you did too much, or not enough.

- Never stop learning, even if it's not something you will ever use. It keeps you humble.

- Validate yourself once in a while.

- Never expect rewards or recognition. Do what is right, simply because it is the right thing to do.

- Do not try to control everything.

Forgiving People

Since so much of our self-esteem is tied up in what the people of our past did or did not do for us, it is important to forgive those who may have harmed us. We often hold onto grudges, and this prevents us from moving forward. Part of having self-esteem is no longer allowing others to control us. If the actions of people in the past still impact the opinion we have of ourselves, then we are still under there control. The main idea of forgiveness is that you have the ability to move on without having to carry a heavy burden any longer. Here is what forgiveness does not mean:

- Condoning harmful behavior.

- Accepting someone back into your life.

- Forgetting the incident or incidents that harmed you.

- Having to talk to the person again in any way.

- You are helping the other person. Of course, this may be a secondary benefit, which is fine.

By forgiving someone, you are accepting the reality that they did something terrible to you, but it no longer has to define you. Forgiveness is 100 percent for your own benefit.

The first step in forgiveness is the willingness to actually forgive someone. Just imagine that the anger you have for someone is a bag of rocks that you have been carrying on your back. After many years, this becomes very exhausting, both physically and mentally. Now, imagine that forgiveness means dropping that bag of rocks forever. You will feel much better when you put down the bag, and you will feel much better once you forgive. When you are ready, then utilize the following steps to help you get past, well, your past.

- Think about the particular incidents that angered you. Accept that they happened and what your feelings were when they did. In order to forgive, you must acknowledge what happened. You cannot just ignore it. This is why forgetting is not part of the process. For example, the incident could have been that your parents were absent and did not pay any attention to you.

- Acknowledge the growth in yourself that happened after the incident occurred. What did it make you learn about yourself and the world? For example, if your parents were absent for much of your life, perhaps it taught you how to be independent and survive on your own. That is a pretty big deal.

- Now think about the other person. The one that actually caused the incident. Realize that they were working from a limited frame of mind and did not have the benefit of hindsight. When they harmed you in some way, they were probably trying to have one of their needs met. Think about what that need may have been, and if it changes your perspective on them. In reference to your parents, maybe they were absent and did not pay attention to you because they were worried about always having food on the table and a roof over your head. This caused them to work incessantly, and when they were home, they were too tired to give you the right amount of attention. It's possible that they hated being absent just as much as you did.

- Finally, say the words, "I forgive you." It is up to you whether you want to tell the person or not. In any event, tell yourself.

Forgiveness will help you put closure on your past so that you can focus on moving forward. This is an important step forward to gaining self-esteem. You will no longer be bound by what happened to you in the past; therefore, you will be free.

Overcoming Trauma

Since trauma plays a major role in a person's self-image, it is important to identify the negative thoughts that will lead to low self-esteem. Once you catch these thoughts, then you can combat them head-on. You may never forget about the trauma, but just like the hurt you received from people of your past, you can keep it from controlling you. The following are a few simple steps you can take to help you improve your negative self-image related to trauma. These practices have been used widely with people suffering from Post Traumatic Stress Disorder.

- Identify your negative thoughts. Once negative thoughts become part of your routine, they can easily slip by without getting caught. Self-monitoring can be a great way of increasing awareness of your thoughts and how they are affecting your mood and behavior. You must do this consciously. You may also sit down at the end of each day and run down what you did. Think about all of the negative thoughts you had, what caused them, and how you reacted. This can also make you more aware of them in the future. We often have specific triggers that affect our mood.

- Once you learn to identify negative thoughts, slow them down. The more you think about negative thoughts, the more intense they become. Therefore, once you identify them, distract yourself by thinking of something else. This is not about avoidance, but taking a step back and reducing the intensity of these thoughts. Often times, we cannot deal with negativity because it becomes so overwhelming. Once we remove ourselves from the situation a little bit, then we can manage things more appropriately.

- After reducing the intensity of your thoughts, it is now time to challenge them. Many times, we accept our thoughts at face value without actually questioning them. As a result, we do not actually know why we are thinking negatively during a certain situation. We just know that we always have. Challenge your thoughts by asking some of the following questions:

  o What evidence is there for having these thoughts?
  o What evidence is there that are against these thoughts?
  o Are there moments when these thoughts have not been true?
  o Do I only have these thoughts when I am sad, angry, or depressed, or do I have them when I am feeling okay, as well?
  o What advice would I give someone else who is also having these thoughts?
  o Is there any type of alternate explanation?

- Counter your negative thoughts further by using positive self-supportive statements. For example, you can tell yourself all of your recent accomplishments, the good qualities you do possess, or positive things you are looking forward to in the future, like starting a new job or taking a vacation. Basically, counter negative thoughts with positive ones. It is beneficial to write some of these down so you can refer to them in the future. When you are drowning in negativity, it can be difficult to come up with positive statements about yourself.

- As a side note, you do not have to use positive self-supportive statements exclusively when you are upset. You can tell them to yourself any time to build up your positivity.

Chapter 4: Changing Our Minds

For the final chapter in this section, we can start focusing on shifting the mindest fully towards high self-esteem. Once this occurs, we must continue to follow the strategies I have gone over to never lose your self-esteem. If you let your guard down, it will happen.

How To Ignore Things

Our self-esteem continues to remain low throughout our lives because we always let things bother us. Many of these things are beyond our control, so we should not pay them any mind. The reason people achieve their lifelong goals is that they don't let their surroundings affect their minds. The following are some ways to ignore what bothers you, so you can keep moving forward while loving yourself.

Stop Comparing Yourself To Others

The bottom line is, you are not someone else, and they are not you. Just because someone else looks great in a dress or suit, does not mean you have to, as well. Also, understand that other people will not look as good as you in certain outfits. Some people will look great all dressed up, while others pull off the casual look better.

If you are not comfortable, then you will never feel right in any situation.

Therefore, do not force yourself into something, simply because other people are doing it. Understand yourself through self-awareness and focus on the things that make you feel good. You can't compare yourself to others, and they can't compare themselves to you. Work on impressing the person in the mirror and no one else.

Ignore Societal Pressure

Have you ever done something because someone you don't like or even know might become impressed, even though they don't actually care about you? If this statement sounds ridiculous, imagine actually living. Oh, wait! Many people are already. This is because they are under some sort of societal pressure to live a certain way, even though most people in society don't matter to them in the long run. To stop allowing this to happen, ask yourself the following questions.

- Who will be responsible after I kill my dreams to produce a fake image, society, or me?
- Are the people around me genuinely concerned about my happiness? If not, then why do I care so much?
- Will the people pressuring me even matter five years from now?
- Am I alone in feeling this societal pressure?

After answering all of these questions, you will realize that your situation is not unique. Many people are pressured by society and trying to hold up a fake image. This means they are not happy because they are not willing to share their true selves. Ultimately, you will be living your own existence, whether you choose it or someone else does.

Start Living In The Present Moment

So many people live in the past, and therefore, their old mistakes still have an impact on their present state of mind. It's time to get over your past. The following are some tips to help you do so.

- Create some physical distance between yourself and the person or situation that is reminding you of your past. This could mean cutting off some close people or physically moving somewhere else.

- Stay busy working and improving yourself, that you have no time to worry about what happened in the past.

- Treat yourself like you would a best friend. We tend to be gentler with others than ourselves.

- Don't shut out negative emotions. Let them flow through you so you can overcome them.

- Don't expect an apology from other people. Even if you were wronged by them, they might not think so. Therefore, move on and accept that they haven't come to terms with anything, but you have.

- Give yourself permission to talk about your pain, even if it's just to yourself. In any event, let it out. Let the past pain escape out of you.

Leverage Your Purpose

This will give your life more meaning. First, leverage your purpose to serve others. Help someone else realize their dreams through your own unique talents. There are many unique ways to do this, including teaching, coaching, and mentoring. Do this on a volunteer basis. Whatever gives purpose to your life, share it with someone else.

Try out these different practices and feel yourself start ignoring all of the noise around you. It is distracting, and you must be able to filter it.

The Mindset Shift

We have gone over many different aspects of the mind and how to change certain thought-processes. What happens with these techniques is a total mindset shift. Instead of your mind being wired to think negatively about everything, including yourself, you will now habitually think in a positive way and understand the values you bring to the world, which are a lot. The goal of all of the previous practices and strategies is to rewire your neural pathways to help change your mindset.

Your mindset was developed over a long period of time, which means the neural pathways you have are build up pretty strong. For this reason, they must be worked on regularly to help break them down and build new ones up. So, do not treat these techniques as a one-and-done cure. They must become a regular part of your lifestyle. Once they are, then you will be amazed at the results you have. When your self-esteem is high, you will:

- Have no problem being yourself.

- Be able to disagree without attacking someone.

- Not be swayed so easily by the opinions of others.

- Be able to articulate your views and be able to defend them appropriately when challenged.

- No longer fear uncertainty.

- Be much more resilient and tough.

- Never need approval from anyone to live your life as you choose.

- Value yourself and have high self-worth, despite what others may think of you.

- Not act like you know everything.

- Be okay with not being perfect.

- Never again let your past define who you are.

Once you go from low to high self-esteem, you will feel like a completely different person. You will still acknowledge your past pain, but it will not control you.

Now That Your Self-Esteem is High

After going through all of the practices, thoughts, and feelings inside of you will be different because you will have effectively restructured your mind. The plan now is to keep revisiting these techniques, so you never fall back into the abyss ever again. Now that your self-esteem is high, you will sense the following beliefs flowing through you.

- No matter what you've done, you are worthy of love. You understand your past mistakes, but will not degrade yourself over them.

- You are not defined by your "stuff." You will enjoy what you have, but your happiness will not be dependent on it.

- You will allow yourself to feel all of your emotions, and not be ashamed of them.

- You won't care if you miss out on things. You will feel okay about staying alone because your company is good enough.

- You will not be worried about what happens to you, because you will be able to respond appropriately, There will be challenges, but the end result will be in your favor.

- You will be doing what you love. You will look forward to every day.

- You will understand that people are judging you based on something within themselves.

- You will never think the world revolves around you. There is a higher power out there greater than anything that exists on Earth. This does not have to be a diety, but it certainly can be for you.

- You will find things to be grateful for every day. Because you are looking, you will find them.

CPSIA information can be obtained
at www.ICGtesting.com
Printed in the USA
BVHW040556110321
602263BV00004B/17